Get Through
FRCA Primary: 710 MCQs

Get Through
FRCA Primary: 710 MCQs

Raja L A Jayaweera MA LLB MBBS DA FRCA
Consultant Anaesthetist, Whittington Hospital, London

Ramanie Jayaweera MBBS FRCA
Provisional Fellow in Paediatric Anaesthesia, Children's Hospital, Westmead, Sydney, Australia

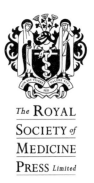

The ROYAL
SOCIETY of
MEDICINE
PRESS Limited

© 2006 Royal Society of Medicine Press Ltd

Reprinted 2007

Published by the Royal Society of Medicine Press Ltd
1 Wimpole Street, London W1G 0AE, UK
Tel: +44 (0)20 7290 2921
Fax: +44 (0)20 7290 2929
Email: publishing@rsm.ac.uk
Website: www.rsmpress.co.uk

British Library Cataloguing in Publication Data
A catalogue record for this book is available from the British Library

ISBN 1-85315-666-3

Distribution in Europe and Rest of World:

Marston Book Services Ltd
PO Box 269
Abingdon
Oxon OX14 4YN, UK
Tel: +44 (0)1235 465500
Fax: +44 (0)1235 465555
Email: direct.order@marston.co.uk

Distribution in the USA and Canada:

Royal Society of Medicine Press Ltd
c/o Bookmasters Inc
30 Amberwood Parkway
Ashland, OH 44805, USA
Tel: +1 800 247 6553/+1 800 266 5564
Fax: +1 419 281 6883
Email: orders@bookmasters.com

Distribution in Australia and New Zealand:

Elsevier Australia
30-52 Smidmore Street
Marrikville NSW 2204, Australia
Tel: +61 2 9349 5811
Fax: +61 2 9349 5911
Email: service@elsevier.com.au

Typeset by Phoenix Photosetting, Chatham, Kent

Printed and bound in Great Britain by Bell & Bain Ltd, Glasgow

Contents

Preface

This book is the effort of two anaesthetists: one has been a teacher of anaesthetics trainees for more than 40 years and, therefore, has some understanding of their needs in respect of the Primary FRCA Examination; the other is a more recent entrant into the specialty of anaesthesia and is aware of the standard of knowledge that is required to pass the Primary FRCA MCQs paper.

The text is divided into two parts: the first, as 'Text Book', consists of 260 MCQs arranged in subject order; the second comprises five 'Test Papers', each with 90 questions. Where appropriate, in addition to the 'True' and 'False' answers, explanatory notes have been included.

From the perception of the authors, trainees find the basic sciences, and in particular physics, the most formidable part of the examination requirements. The continuing and rapid advances in these sciences, and the imperative to apply this new information in their anaesthetic practice, make a mere 'upgrade' of undergraduate knowledge inadequate to meet the requirements for success in the Primary FRCA Examination. To meet this need, the authors have essentially confined their attention to physiology, pharmacology, clinical chemistry and physics. They have chosen to leave clinical anaesthesia relatively untouched because they are of the opinion that trainee anaesthetists find examination questions on that section less difficult than the basic sciences.

Raja L A Jayaweera
Ramanie Jayaweera

Abbreviations

ACE	angiotensin-converting enzyme
AcH	acetyl choline
ACTH	adenocorticotropic hormone
ADH	antidiuretic hormone
AIDS	acquired immune deficiency syndrome
ALA	d aminolaevulinic acid
AMP	adenosine monophosphate
AMPA	α-amino-3-hydroxy-5-methylioxazole-4-propionic acid
ANP	atrial natriuretic peptide
APL	adjustable pressure-limiting valve
ASD	atrial septal defect
ATP	adenosine triphosphate
AV	atrioventricular
BBB	blood–brain barrier
BCE	butryl cholinesterase
BCDFE	bromochlorodifluoroethylene
BG	blood-gas
BMR	basal metabolic rate
BP	blood pressure
Camp	cyclic adenosine 3′-5′-monophosphate
CBF	cerebral blood flow
CBG	corticosteroid-binding globulin
CGS	centimetre gram second
CMR	cerebral metabolic rate
CNS	central nervous system
CO	cardiac output
COMT	catechol O-methyl transferase
COPD	chronic obstructive pulmonary disease
COX	cyclor-oxygenase
CPAP	continuous positive airway pressure
CSF	cerebrospinal fluid
CTZ	chemoreceptor trigger zone
CV	cardiovascular
CVP	central venous pressure
DBS	double-burst stimulation
DPG	diphosphoglycerate
ECF	extracellular fluid (compartment)
ECH	electrocardiogram
ECT	electro-convulsive therapy
EDRF	endothelium-derived relaxing factor
EEG	electroencephalogram
EMF	electro-motive force
EMR	electromagnetic radiations
ET-1	endothelin-1
EW	Edinber–Westphal nucleus
FCG	French catheter gauge
FFP	fresh frozen plasma
FRC	functional residual capacity

GABA	gamma-aminobutyric acid
GI	gastrointestinal
GLUT	glucose transporter
GMP	guanosine monophosphate
GST	glutathione-S-transferase
HbA1c	glycosylated haemoglobin
HDLs	high-density lipoproteins
HESs	heta-starches
HPV	hypoic pulmonary vasoconstriction
ICF	intracellular fluid compartment
IDLs	intermediate-density lipoproteins
IR	infrared
IT	interstitial compartment
KOH	potassium hydroxide
LA	local anaesthetic
LDLs	low-density lipoproteins
LED	light-emitting diode
LMW	low-molecular weight protein
LT	lung-thorax
MAC	minimum alveolar concentration
MAO	monoamine oxidase
MRI	magnetic resonance imaging
MW	molecular weight
NAChK	nicotinic acetylcholine receptor
NADPH	nicotinamide adenine diphosphonucleotide
NCARCs	(nicotinic acetylcholine receptors)
NM	neuromuscular
NMBAs	neuromuscular blocking agents
NMDA	N-methyl D-aspartate
NMJs	neuromuscular junctions
NO	nitric oxide
NOP	nociceptor orphanin Q peptide
NSAIDs	non-steroidal anti-inflammatory drugs
OCPs	oral contraceptives
OSA	obstructive sleep apnoea
PAF	platelet-activating factor
PONV	postoperative nausea and vomiting
PG_2	prostaglandin$_2$
PNS	peripheral nerve stimulator
PVR	pulmonary vascular resistance
Pta	prothrombin activator
REM	rapid eye movement
RMS	root mean square
RQ	respiratory quotient
SA	sino-atrial
SELV	safety extra low voltage equipment
SGLT	sodium-glucose transporter
SRSA	substance of anaphylaxis
SSRIs	selective serotonin re-uptake inhibitors
STP	standard temperature and pressure
SVR	systemic vascular resistance
SWG	steel wire gauge

TOF	Train-of-Four
TXA	thromboxane
US	ultrasound
VC	vital capacity
VF	ventricular fibrillation
VIP	vasoactive intestinal peptide
VLDLs	very low-density lipoproteins
VPC	volumes per cent
VSCC	voltage sensitive Ca channels

Anatomy

1　**The following statements are true:**

　a. All the extrinsic muscles of the eye except the lateral rectus are supplied by the oculomotor nerve.
　b. Of the cervical spinal nerves, the first is the only one that has no cutaneous distribution.
　c. The whole of the cutaneous supply of the head comes from the trigeminal nerve and the cervical spinal nerves.
　d. Of the arteries arising from the Circle of Willis only the anterior communicating artery is unpaired.
　e. The thoracic segments of the spinal cord are the only ones that possess an intermediolateral horn.

2　**The following cranial nerves are solely motor in function:**

　a. Oculomotor nerve.
　b. Abducens nerve.
　c. Lingual nerve.
　d. Glossopharyngeal nerve.
　e. Spinal accessory nerve.

3　**The vagus nerves:**

　a. Account for more than half the activity of the parasympathetic nervous system.
　b. Have more sensory fibres than motor fibres.
　c. Leave the skull through the foramen magnum.
　d. Enter the abdomen through the aortic opening in the diaphragm.
　e. Together supply the large intestine as far as the sigmoid colon.

4　**In the case of the larynx:**

　a. It extends from the level of the 2nd cervical vertebra to that of the 7th.
　b. All its intrinsic muscles receive their motor supply from the recurrent laryngeal nerve.
　c. Its mucous membrane is entirely columnar ciliated in nature.
　d. Its sensory supply is solely from the recurrent laryngeal nerves.
　e. Its arterial blood supply is solely from the superior thyroid artery.

5   **In the case of the lungs:**

a. The cervical pleura ascends above the level of the medial third of the clavicle.
b. The oblique fissure of the lung starts posteriorly at the level of the 5th thoracic vertebra.
c. The horizontal fissure (of the right lung) ends anteriorly at the 4th chondrosternal junction.
d. At the midpoint of quiet inspiration the lower border of the lung ends posteriorly at the level of the 8th rib adjacent to the vertebral column.
e. At rest the lung hila are at the level of the 2nd to 4th costal cartilages.

6   **The following statements are true:**

a. The cords of the brachial plexus are formed solely from the ventral rami of C5–8 and T1.
b. The venous drainage of the heart is entirely into the coronary (venous) sinus.
c. The whole of the cranial parasympathetic outflow originates in nuclei in the medulla oblongata.
d. Every cervical spinal nerve provides a cutaneous supply to the head and neck.
e. Every spinal nerve receives a grey ramus communicans from the sympathetic outflow.

7   **The phrenic nerve:**

a. Arises from cervical roots 3–5.
b. Is purely motor in function.
c. Is the sole motor supply to the diaphragm.
d. Descends on the posterior aspect of the scalenus anterior muscle.
e. Enters the thorax behind the subclavian artery.

8   **In the classification of nerve fibres:**

a. Type A fibres are the typical myelinated fibres of spinal nerves.
b. Type C fibres conduct impulses at high velocity.
c. δ -type fibres are responsible for temperature and crude touch sensations.
d. γ -type fibres are the slowest-conducting fibres.
e. All the postganglionic autonomic fibres are of Type C.

9   Concerning the anatomy of the heart:

    a. The right coronary artery arises from the right posterior aortic sinus.
    b. The left coronary artery gives rise to the circumflex artery.
    c. The Thebesian vessels drain directly into all four chambers of the heart.
    d. The sympathetic supply is from the intermediolateral horns of the middle thoracic segments.
    e. The sinoatrial node receives its parasympathetic supply from the left vagus nerve.

10   **The following statements are true with respect to the autonomic nervous system:**

    a. The vagus nerve conveys afferent pain fibres.
    b. Postganglionic sympathetic nerves are more likely to be myelinated than non-myelinated.
    c. All postganglionic sympathetic nerve terminals have adrenaline or noradrenaline as their neurotransmitter.
    d. Some preganglionic sympathetic fibres directly innervate their target organs.
    e. The cranial parasympathetic outflow arises solely in the medulla oblongata.

11   The cell membrane:

   a. Is about 5–10 angstrom thick.
   b. Is an amphoteric structure.
   c. Is symmetrical in nature.
   d. Is a fluid mosaic.
   e. In its behaviour is micelle like.

12   The Na^+–K^+–ATPase pump:

   a. Is an electrogenic pump.
   b. Is present in all cells of the body.
   c. Is the prime determinant of the water content of the intracellular fluid compartment.
   d. Is the basis of nerve activity associated with transmission of impulses throughout the nervous system.
   e. Is the molecular mechanism by which digoxin exerts its positive cardiac inotropic action.

13   The following are passive transmembranal transport processes:

   a. Bulk flow.
   b. Solvent drag.
   c. Simple diffusion.
   d. Facilitated diffusion.
   e. Pinocytosis.

14   Simple diffusion of drugs across membranes:

   a. Occurs solely through the lipid bilayer.
   b. Shows first-order kinetics.
   c. Is subject to a 'ceiling effect'.
   d. In rate is directly proportional to the square root of the concentration gradient.
   e. In rate is directly proportional to the square root of the molecular weight of the solute.

15   Carrier-mediated transport of drugs:

   a. Is effected by intrinsic membrane proteins.
   b. Is generally unidirectional.
   c. Always requires expenditure of cellular energy in its own right.
   d. Can occur against a concentration gradient.
   e. Is subject to a ceiling effect.

16   The following are common to facilitated diffusion and primary active transport:

a. They both need a carrier protein.
b. They can both occur against a concentration gradient.
c. They are both subject to a ceiling effect.
d. They are both temperature dependent.
e. They are both utilised as forms of transport of glucose into cells.

17   G protein-coupled receptors:

a. Constitute the largest family of cell surface receptors.
b. Possess the property of pleiotropy.
c. Depend for their activity on the dissociation of the G protein into its constitutive subunits.
d. Have a significant role in fast synaptic transmission between excitable cells.
e. Are the predominant receptor category for anaesthetic drug action.

18   AMPA (α-amino-3-hydroxy-5-methylioxazole-4-propionic acid) receptors:

a. Are a category of metabotropic receptors.
b. Are a type of fast excitatory transmitter in the central nervous system (CNS).
c. Are receptors whose channels are permeable to cations.
d. Generally have a high affinity for glutamate.
e. On hyperactivation can bring about nerve cell death.

19   The Embden–Meyerhof (glycolytic) metabolic pathway:

a. Is an amphibolic pathway.
b. Occurs in the mitochondria.
c. Necessarily requires oxygen for its functioning.
d. Releases CO_2 as one of its by-products.
e. Produces about half the ATP as does the Krebs tricarboxylic acid cycle.

20   The following are attributes common to nitric oxide and prostacyclin:

a. They are both autacoids.
b. They both relax underlying smooth muscle of endothelium on its abluminal side.
c. They both work via the guanylyl cyclase mechanism.
d. Their actions last for only a few seconds.
e. They both work equally effectively in producing vasodilatation, even in the presence of endothelial damage.

21   Myelin:

a. Has a higher lipid content than cell cytoplasm.
b. Has a higher refractive index than the cell cytosol.
c. Is electrically insulating.
d. Gives a grey colour to the nerves.
e. Is found in profusion in sheaths of axons within the CNS.

22   Nitric oxide:

a. Is exactly the same as endothelium-derived relaxing factor (EDRF).
b. Is enzyme dependent for its production.
c. Is released as a result of shear stress on endothelium wall cells.
d. Requires combination with a haem-containing domain to bring about its action.
e. Has a half-life of about 3–4 minutes.

23   Inhaled nitric oxide:

a. Is a lipophilic gas.
b. Causes pulmonary vasodilatation as well as systemic vasodilatation.
c. Is inactivated by haemoglobin.
d. Has been known to cause methaemoglobinaemia.
e. Can in overdose produce toxic effects from being converted to other oxides of nitrogen.

24   In the case of the sympathetic nervous system:

a. Both pre- and postganglionic fibres are myelinated.
b. Myelinated fibres are grey in appearance.
c. Pre-ganglionic fibres originate in the anterior horn cells of the spinal cord.
d. Postganglionic fibres innervate the adrenal medulla.
e. Its distribution to the head and neck arises in thoracic segments 1–4 of the cord.

25   In the case of the parasympathetic nervous system:

a. Its pre- and postganglionic fibres are of approximately equal length.
b. Its cranial outflow originates entirely in the medulla oblongata.
c. More than half of its nerve fibres are in the vagus nerves.
d. Its transmitter substance at both pre- and postganglionic sites is acetylcholine.
e. It provides fibres to the cardiac ventricles in equal measure with the sympathetic nervous system.

26 The following are paired autonomic sympathetic ganglia:

a. Stellate ganglion.
b. Coeliac ganglion.
c. Superior mesenteric ganglion.
d. Ganglion impar.
e. Inferior mesenteric ganglion.

27 The dominant autonomic tone in the following is adrenergic rather than cholinergic:

a. Activity of the sino-atrial node.
b. Arteriolar constriction.
c. Bronchomotor activity.
d. Gastrointestinal function.
e. Liver glycogenolysis.

28 Sympathetic agonism will lead to:

a. Vasoconstriction of the gut.
b. Bronchodilatation.
c. Liver glycogenolysis.
d. Insulin release from the pancreas.
e. Inhibition of anti-diuretic hormone (ADH) release from the posterior pituitary.

29 Acetylcholine:

a. Is a quaternary ammonium compound.
b. Is a muscarinic agonist.
c. Dilates virtually all blood vessels.
d. Causes hyperpolarisation of the membrane of the sino-atrial node.
e. Is released on stimulation of carotid and aortic body chemoreceptors.

30 Adrenaline (Epinephrine)

a. Is a substituted catecholamine.
b. Is a quaternary ammonium compound.
c. Is producible from noradrenaline (norepinephrine) by removal of a –CH$_3$ group.
d. Constitutes about 25% of the catecholamine secretion of the adrenal medulla.
e. Is the predominant agonist at postganglionic sympathetic α nerve endings.

31   α_2-adrenergic receptors:

a. Are usually pre-synaptic in location.
b. Are found in high density in the cerebral cortex.
c. Also exist on cholinergic nerve terminals.
d. Have clonidine as their prototype agonist.
e. Have prazosin as their prototype antagonist.

32   The following are manifestations of adrenergic inhibition:

a. Hypokalaemia.
b. Hyperglycaemia.
c. Rise in free fatty acids in the plasma.
d. Ptosis.
e. Postoperative ileus.

33   The following β-adrenergic blockers possess intrinsic cardiac sympathomimetic activity:

a. Acebutolol.
b. Atenolol.
c. Esmolol.
d. Pindolol.
e. Propranolol.

34   Pupillary dilatation:

a. Is a manifestation of α_1-adrenergic agonism.
b. Is mediated through increased activity at the Edinger–Westphal nucleus.
c. Is the usual outcome of stellate ganglion block.
d. Is enhanced by pilocarpine.
e. Is diminished by ecothiopate.

35   H_1 receptor antagonists:

a. Are generally effective in the management of asthma.
b. Generally also have anti-muscarinic actions.
c. Are of little use in the management of acute anaphylaxis.
d. Have a pronounced depressant effect on ventilatory drive in usual clinical dosage.
e. Cannot prevent the hypotensive effect of histamine.

36   Concerning endothelium-derived relaxing factor (EDRF):

   a. It is exactly the same thing as nitric oxide.
   b. It acts via formation of adenosine monophosphate (AMP) from adenosine triphosphate.
   c. Its release is inhibited by raised levels of calcium ions.
   d. It inhibits platelet aggregation.
   e. It is regarded as the mediator in the vasodilator effect of sodium nitroprusside.

37   Concerning brown adipose tissue ('brown fat'):

   a. It is only found in infants.
   b. It has a regular location in the interscapular region.
   c. It has a richer blood supply compared to 'white' fat.
   d. It has a rich α-adrenergic innervation.
   e. Its activity is the basis of non-shivering thermogenesis.

38   The respiratory quotient:

   a. Is a 'dimensionless entity'.
   b. Is a 'steady-state' measurement.
   c. Is higher when the substrate is carbohydrate rather than fat.
   d. Is higher for cardiac muscle metabolism than for brain cell metabolism.
   e. During severe exercise can attain a level more than twice that at rest.

39   Zinc is an integral element in the structure and activity of the following enzymes:

   a. Alcohol dehydrogenase.
   b. Butyryl cholinesterase.
   c. Carbonic anhydrase.
   d. Cyclo-oxygenase.
   e. Protein kinase C.

40   Ethyl alcohol:

   a. Is absorbed from the alimentary tract by passive diffusion.
   b. Undergoes first-pass metabolism in gastric mucosal cells.
   c. Is usually subject to zero-order kinetics.
   d. Has a diuretic effect unrelated to fluid intake.
   e. For the same dose gives a higher blood concentration in women solely because of their lower percentage body water content.

41   Ethyl alcohol:

a. Inhibits glucogenesis.
b. Increases the likelihood of lactic acidosis.
c. Inhibits oxidation of fatty acids.
d. Causes accumulation of acetyl co-enzyme A.
e. Decreases the amount of NO synthase.

42   In the case of atrial natriuretic peptide (ANP):

a. It is a nonapeptide.
b. It is secreted solely by the atria.
c. Its release occurs in response to volume receptor activity.
d. It produces its effect by activation of adenylyl cyclase.
e. It inhibits aldosterone release mainly by a primary action on the adrenal cortex.

43   Water:

a. Is a polar substance.
b. Has a high surface tension.
c. Has a low vapour pressure.
d. Has a high specific heat capacity.
e. Has a low heat of vaporisation.

44   Of the four crystalloid IV solutions (Hartmann's solution, N-Saline, Glucose–Saline and 5% Glucose):

a. Hartmann's solution has a pH nearest that of the extracellular fluid.
b. N-saline is the most acidic.
c. 5% glucose has the highest 'free water' content.
d. Glucose–saline has one-fifth the sodium content of Hartmann's solution.
e. They all have a calculated osmolarity of about 280–290 mmol/L of solution.

45   One litre of Hartmann's solution:

a. Has 29 mmol of sodium bicarbonate as buffer.
b. Contains 2 milliequivalents of calcium.
c. Has about 200 mg of potassium.
d. Usually contains a trace of sodium hydroxide.
e. On rapid IV infusion in a normal standard-size adult person, will also distribute itself into the interstitial compartment mainly as the result of an osmolar gradient.

46. **Dextrans:**

   a. Are straight chain polysaccharides of glucose.
   b. Improve peripheral blood flow by causing vasodilatation.
   c. Impair platelet adhesiveness.
   d. Impair Factor VIII activity.
   e. Can interfere with blood cross-matching.

47 **Haemaccel:**

   a. Contains gelatin with an average molecular weight of c. 60 kDa.
   b. Is presented in half-litre packs as a 7.5% w/v solution.
   c. Contains chloride in a concentration comparable with that of normal saline.
   d. Contains calcium.
   e. Has a pH near that of whole blood.

48 **Gelofusine:**

   a. Is succinylated gelatin.
   b. Is 4% w/v preparation.
   c. Has a pH near that of plasma.
   d. Contains sodium and chloride in concentrations comparable with those of plasma.
   e. Contains no added calcium.

49 **In the case of hydroxyethyl starches:**

   a. They are straight chain compounds.
   b. The higher their substitution index the lower their solubility.
   c. The higher their substitution index the longer their intravascular half-life.
   d. They have a higher water-binding capacity than the gelatins.
   e. The higher the weight-averaged molecular weight of the preparation the greater the interference with clotting factors.

50 **The plasma sodium concentration:**

   a. Accounts for about 40–50% of the plasma osmolarity.
   b. Is of a slightly higher value compared with that in the interstitial compartment.
   c. Is the prime determinant of the amount of extracellular water.
   d. Is the main factor determining the secretion of anti-diuretic hormone.
   e. Is about the same as the sodium concentration of normal saline.

51 **In the case of the secretions of the alimentary tract:**

a. Saliva is always hypotonic to plasma.
b. Gastric juice is the only one that does not have bicarbonate.
c. Pancreatic juice has the highest pH.
d. Gall bladder bile has a higher bicarbonate concentration than pancreatic juice.
e. None of the secretions has a chloride content above that of the plasma.

52. **The following are features regarding the absorption of sodium in the gastrointestinal (GI) tract:**

a. Sodium absorption occurs along the entire length of the intestine.
b. The net rate of sodium absorption is lowest in the jejunum.
c. Sodium absorption requires a significant net concentration gradient across the luminal interface.
d. Sodium absorption enhances the absorption of glucose and amino acids.
e. Active sodium absorption occurs only at the basolateral membrane interface.

53 **The following physiological changes occur when a normal adult drinks 2 L of water rapidly:**

a. There will be loss of about 25% of the volume in the faeces.
b. Absorption of the water in the gut will take place by active transfer at the luminal surface.
c. An almost immediate diuresis is initiated as a result of posterior pituitary activity.
d. Movement of water at the basal membrane of gut cells is still dependent on the active transfer of sodium.
e. A substantial fraction of the water will enter the general intracellular fluid compartment.

54 **The anion gap:**

a. Is the difference between the 'measured cations and the measured anions in the plasma'.
b. Increases when organic anions accumulate.
c. Is greater when there is an acidosis from bicarbonate loss or chloride excess.
d. Is lower with hypoalbuminaemia.
e. Is greater when there is a fall in unmeasured cations.

55   **In the case of a blood gas analysis result, which accurately reflects the patient's clinical chemistry:**

   a. The presence of a normal pH rules out any acid-base disturbance.
   b. A normal paO_2 indicates normoventilation.
   c. A low paO_2 and a raised $paCO_2$ are indicative of underventilation.
   d. A raised bicarbonate necessarily indicates a metabolic alkalosis.
   e. A low pCO_2 and a normal bicarbonate necessarily indicate a respiratory alkalosis with metabolic compensation.

56   **In a primary acute respiratory acidosis:**

   a. There is a rise in the standard bicarbonate.
   b. The haemoglobin oxygen dissociation curve is shifted to the left.
   c. There is a rapid fall in urinary pH.
   d. There is increased urinary excretion of chloride.
   e. Sodium bicarbonate is of use in correcting the acidosis.

57   **The HCO_3'/H_2CO_3 system is a useful buffer system because:**

   a. Its pKa is very near that of the plasma.
   b. It is present in large amounts in the extracellular fluid.
   c. It is the only buffer system that links the two acid-excreting organs of the body.
   d. Its ingredients are rapidly convertible to a non-ionised and easily excretable product.
   e. It is the only buffer whose constituents are conveniently measurable in clinical practice.

58   **Carbon dioxide is carried in the blood as:**

   a. Dissolved CO_2 in the plasma.
   b. Carboxyhaemoglobin.
   c. Carbonic acid.
   d. Bicarbonate.
   e. Carbamate.

59   **The combination of oxygen with haemoglobin:**

   a. Is a process of oxidation.
   b. Is a homotropic negative cooperative effect.
   c. Is enhanced by 2,3 diphosphoglycerate.
   d. Leads to a progressive decrease in the number of haemoglobin molecules in the 'relaxed' state.
   e. Is a phenomenon analogous to that which occurs with many allosteric enzymes.

60   It is the globin moiety of haemoglobin:

   a. That is responsible for the red colour of haemoglobin.
   b. That is responsible for its acid-base buffering ability.
   c. That combines with CO_2 in the latter's carriage in the blood.
   d. That is responsible for the biochemical aberrations that give
      rise to thalassaemia.
   e. That, when abnormal, gives rise to porphyria.

61   The combination of haemoglobin with each of the following is
       enzyme dependent:

   a. Oxygen.
   b. Carbon dioxide.
   c. Carbon monoxide.
   d. Nitric oxide.
   e. Glucose to form glycosylated haemoglobin (HbA1c).

62   Patients suffering from the following haemoglobinopathies are
       likely to have a higher P_{50} than normal adult haemoglobin A:

   a. Thalassaemia.
   b. Methaemoglobinaemia.
   c. Sulphaemoglobinaemia.
   d. Carboxyhaemoglobinaemia.
   e. Sickle cell disease.

63   An arterial haemoglobin oxygen saturation of 96% correctly
       indicates that:

   a. The arterial pO_2 is about 13–14 kPa.
   b. The arterial pCO_2 is within normal limits.
   c. There is enough oxygen in the patient's blood for basal
      oxygen needs.
   d. There is no tissue hypoxia.
   e. There cannot be any significant level of carboxyhaemoglobin
      in the blood.

64   2,3 diphosphoglycerate (2,3 DPG):

   a. Is formed from 2,3 diphosphoglyceraldehyde.
   b. Is a by-product of the activity of the Krebs tricarboxylic cycle.
   c. Is a highly charged ion.
   d. Is bound to the α chain of the haemoglobin molecule.
   e. Is present in a concentration of 1 molecule per haem moiety of
      each haemoglobin molecule.

65   The effective viscosity of whole blood is dependent on:

a. Haematocrit.
b. Fibrinogen content.
c. Temperature.
d. Vessel radius.
e. Linear velocity of blood flow.

66   Concerning the ABO blood group system:

a. The A and B antigens are inherited as mendelian dominants.
b. The A and B antigens are mainly glycoproteins.
c. The antibodies are predominantly IgD and IgE immunoglobulins.
d. Blood group type O persons have an H antigen.
e. When there is an antigen–antibody reaction it is the antibodies of the donor blood that combine with the antigen of the recipient red cells.

67   The following blood diseases are usually inherited as autosomal dominants:

a. Von Willebrand's disease.
b. Haemophilia A.
c. Haemophilia B.
d. Factor VII deficiency.
e. Factor X deficiency.

68   The formation of carbaminohaemoglobin:

a. Occurs when carbon monoxide combines with haemoglobin.
b. Results from combination of the relevant substance at the haem moiety of the haemoglobin molecule.
c. Is dependent on the presence of an enzyme in the red cells.
d. Accounts for most of the transportation of the relevant agent in the blood.
e. Is concurrently associated with the Hamburger phenomenon.

69   In the case of methaemoglobinaemia:

a. It can sometimes be associated with infection with *Pneumocystis carinii*.
b. It has been known to follow Bier's block (IV local anaesthesia).
c. It usually does not produce symptoms at a concentration less than 20%.
d. When present it can vitiate the accuracy of conventional SpO_2 oximetry.
e. Methylene blue given for treatment can sometimes worsen the clinical state.

70   The following dyshaemoglobinaemias cause a shift of the haemoglobin dissociation curve to the left:

    a. Carboxyhaemoglobin.
    b. Methaemoglobin.
    c. Sulphaemoglobin.
    d. Fetal haemoglobin.
    e. Sickle cell haemoglobin S.

71   The following changes occur in transfusion blood (containing no additives apart from anticoagulant) stored at 4°C:

    a. Fall in pH.
    b. Rise in serum potassium.
    c. Fall in plasma sodium.
    d. Rise in level of 2,3 diphosphoglycerate.
    e. Fall in level of Factor VIII.

72   **Fresh-frozen plasma:**

    a. Contains all the plasma proteins.
    b. Contains all the clotting factors.
    c. Generally increases level of clotting factors by about 20–30% in the adult per 'unit' of transfused FFP.
    d. Carries the same infection risk as whole blood.
    e. Can only be given safely after ABO compatibility has been ensured.

73   **Platelets:**

    a. Cannot reproduce.
    b. Have a lifespan the same as leucocytes.
    c. Contain actin and myosin similar to those found in skeletal muscle cells.
    d. Contain adenosine diphosphate.
    e. Form leukotrienes.

74   **Platelet concentrate for transfusion:**

    a. Must be stored at room temperature to prevent loss of activity.
    b. Is indicated for thrombocytopenia resulting from immune destruction of platelets.
    c. Must be rendered ABO compatible prior to transfusion.
    d. May be stored up to 24 hours before use.
    e. When given in support for splenectomy for idiopathic thrombocytopenic purpura, ought to be given just prior to commencement of surgery.

75   Concerning the blood coagulation cascade:

   a. It is a positive feedback mechanism.
   b. Its rate-limiting factor is the conversion of prothrombin to thrombin.
   c. The prothrombin to thrombin conversion is accelerated by platelet activity.
   d. The role of calcium is solely that of converting prothrombin to thrombin.
   e. Thrombin's essential role is the conversion of fibrinogen to fibrin monomers.

76   Vitamin K:

   a. Is a fat-soluble vitamin.
   b. Is formed in the colon by bacteria.
   c. Is physiologically active in the cytosol of hepatocytes.
   d. Is required to decarboxylate glutamine moieties of coagulation factors to render them active.
   e. Is inactivated by warfarin by being prevented from undergoing oxidation.

77   The following usually prolong the action of warfarin:

   a. Hypoproteinaemia.
   b. Chronic alcohol ingestion but without alcoholic cirrhosis.
   c. Pregnancy.
   d. Orally administered antibiotics.
   e. Parenteral cephalosporins.

Cardiovascular physiology

78   In the case of the heart under normal conditions:

a. Its left ventricle behaves as a constant pressure generator rather than a constant flow generator.
b. It expends almost equal amounts of energy for 'volume-pressure work' as for accelerating blood to its velocity of ejection through the aortic and pulmonary valves (kinetic work).
c. Both ventricles contract like bellows.
d. Both right and left ventricles contract simultaneously.
e. Both right and left ventricular ejection phases are of equal duration.

79   In the cardiac muscle action potential:

a. The upstroke is associated with an influx of sodium.
b. The early rapid repolarisation is associated with chloride influx.
c. The plateau phase is the result of activity of slow calcium channels.
d. Phase 3 is the 'final repolarisation phase'.
e. The 'diastolic depolarisation phase' is dependent solely on potassium conductivity of cell membrane.

80   The isovolumic relaxation phase of the cardiac cycle:

a. Lasts from aortic valve closure to mitral valve opening.
b. Is concurrent with ventricular depolarisation.
c. Is energy dependent.
d. Is accompanied by a precipitous fall in intraventricular pressure.
e. Makes no contribution to ventricular filling.

81   In the case of innervation of the heart:

a. Both sympathetic and parasympathetic innervation are found with about equal intensity in all four chambers.
b. The cardiac muscarinic receptors are of the M_1 type.
c. The cardiac sympathetic fibres originate in spinal segments T5–8.
d. The sympathetic fibres relay in the stellate ganglion before reaching the heart.
e. Beta 2-adrenergic receptors are mainly confined to the ventricles.

82   The following hormones are secreted by cardiomyocytes:

a. Atrial natriuretic peptide.
b. Aldosterone.
c. Adrenomedullin.
d. Angiotensin II.
e. Glucagon.

83   An increase in the length of cardiac ventricular muscle fibres will usually lead to the following:

a. Increased force of contraction of the ventricle.
b. Increase in the ejection fraction.
c. Stimulation of aortic sinus activity.
d. Inhibition of carotid body activity.
e. Activation of the Bainbridge reflex.

84   The transplanted heart:

a. May show two P-waves on the ECG.
b. Has a high-normal cardiac output.
c. Has a decreased response to catecholamines.
d. Undergoes the highest degree of rejection in the second post-transplantation year.
e. Has a tendency to silent ischaemia.

85   In the normal jugular venous pulse:

a. The a-wave results from closure of the tricuspid valve.
b. The v-wave is almost synchronous with the first heart sound.
c. A 'cannon wave' is an exaggerated c-wave.
d. The pulse waves are attenuated in constrictive pericarditis.
e. The height of the pulse is correctly measured from the Angle of Louis.

86   In the case of the pressure wave of the arterial pulse:

a. It accompanies the pulsatile blood flow that produces it.
b. It becomes more peaked in its graphic display form with increasing distance from the heart.
c. It has a velocity of transmission greater in the aorta than in the arterioles.
d. Its volume is a reliable indicator of the amount of blood flow in the arterial system.
e. It can be relied upon as a reasonable indicator of pulse pressure.

87   When measuring arterial blood pressure by the indirect method using a mercury column and an air-inflated cuff bladder around the upper arm, falsely higher values are more likely to occur:

a. If the arm is held raised above shoulder level.
b. When the forearm and hand muscles are not relaxed.
c. If the mercury reservoir is positioned below cuff level.
d. When cuff width is more than 50% of the arm diameter.
e. If the patient is bradycardic rather than tachycardic.

88   Other things being equal, turbulence from blood flow is more likely:

a. In the aorta than in the arterioles.
b. With a higher cardiac output than with a lower cardiac output.
c. With a higher haematocrit than a lower haematocrit.
d. In a stenotic vessel than in a non-stenosed vessel.
e. With plasma flow than with the flow of water.

89   Compared with the carotid sinus baroreceptors, the aortic sinus baroreceptors:

a. Have a higher threshold for activating the static response.
b. Have a lower threshold for eliciting the dynamic response.
c. Have a higher 'saturation point' when responding to pressure increases.
d. Are more sensitive to the rate of pressure change.
e. Respond less effectively to a decrease in pressure than an increase in pressure (over the same pressure range).

90   In relation to the brain, heart, kidneys, liver and adrenal glands:

a. The brain has the highest oxygen consumption in relation to its mass.
b. The heart has the highest percentage of blood flow in diastole compared with systole.
c. The adrenals have the highest blood flow per unit mass of tissue.
d. The kidneys receive the biggest fraction of the resting cardiac output.
e. The liver has the highest percentage oxygen extraction, i.e. oxygen uptake/oxygen input ratio.

91 **Cardiac muscle differs from skeletal muscle in the following respects:**

   a. It is not striated, while skeletal muscle is.
   b. It possesses 'gap junctions', which skeletal muscle does not.
   c. Its action potential involves two types of ion channel, skeletal muscle does not.
   d. It is capable of a greater maximum force of contraction than skeletal muscle.
   e. It has a much slower velocity of impulse conduction.

92 **Aortic stenosis:**

   a. Is the commonest cardiac valvular lesion in the UK.
   b. Is most commonly caused by rheumatic fever.
   c. Shows symptoms early in its pathogenesis.
   d. Has an increasing incidence with age.
   e. Has a higher anaesthetic morbidity and mortality than any other cardiac valvular disease.

93 **Atrial septal defect:**

   a. Is one of the commonest cardiac malformations.
   b. Is often symptomatic in childhood.
   c. Shows a regular sinus rhythm (rsR) pattern in right chest leads.
   d. Is associated with long-term survival.
   e. Has less than 1% operative mortality for elective repair of uncomplicated ASD.

94 **Hypoxic pulmonary vasoconstriction:**

   a. Is a phenomenon present in all mammalian species.
   b. Occurs independent of the nervous system.
   c. Cannot occur in the absence of an intact pulmonary endothelium.
   d. Occurs in the fetus in utero.
   e. Is augmented by acidosis.

95 **The haemoglobin oxygen saturation of the blood in the following is usually lower than that of mixed venous blood:**

   a. (Internal) jugular venous bulb.
   b. Coronary (venous) sinus.
   c. Hepatic vein.
   d. Renal vein.
   e. Femoral vein.

96   **In the normal healthy young adult at rest:**

a. The anatomical dead space is about the same as the physiological dead space.
b. The alveolar pO_2 is nearly the same as the arterial pO_2.
c. The plasma bicarbonate is approximately the same as the standard bicarbonate.
d. The blood flow through the liver per unit mass is the same as cerebral blood flow per unit mass.
e. The total cardiac oxygen consumption is nearly the same as the total cerebral oxygen consumption.

97   **Under resting conditions the heart:**

a. Has a higher blood flow per unit mass than has the liver.
b. Has a higher oxygen consumption per unit mass than has the brain.
c. Uses a higher amount of glucose as a percentage of its total metabolic substrate than do red blood cells.
d. Requires a higher energy requirement than the work of breathing.
e. Consume a greater percentage of basal energy than does respiratory effort.

98   The anatomical dead space:

a. Extends up to but does not include the alveoli.
b. Is normally about 2–3 ml/kg irrespective of the size of the subject.
c. Relative to tidal volume is greater in the neonate compared with the adult.
d. Is reduced by about 50% on orotracheal intubation.
e. Can be determined by simple spirometry.

99   The following can be determined by direct measurement by simple spirometry:

a. Vital capacity.
b. Anatomical dead space.
c. Residual volume.
d. Physiological dead space.
e. Expiratory reserve volume.

100 During normal quiet spontaneous ventilation in the healthy adult:

a. The anatomical and physiological dead spaces are about equal in volume.
b. A pressure gradient of about 5 cm water is sufficient to maintain adequate gas exchange.
c. The pressure gradient per se takes the tidal gases only as far as the terminal bronchioles.
d. The greatest resistance to gas flow occurs in the smallest bronchioles.
e. About 10–15% of the body's basal energy expenditure is in relation to the work of breathing.

101 In the erect position:

a. Normally, blood flow in the apex of the lung occurs throughout the cardiac cycle.
b. Blood flow in the lung apex is increased during continuous positive airway pressure (CPAP).
c. In Zone 2 systolic pressure > diastolic pressure > alveolar pressure.
d. In Zone 3 pulmonary capillary pressure drops below intra-alveolar pressure.
e. During exercise the whole of lung blood flow is of Zone 3 pattern.

102   **The lung alveoli are normally able to remain dry because:**

a. Pulmonary capillary hydrostatic pressure is low compared with systemic capillary pressure.
b. The interstitial pressure is negative relative to that of the surrounding areas.
c. The lymphatics maintain a slight negative pressure in the pulmonary interstitium.
d. The alveolar epithelium is extremely efficient in preventing fluid leaking out from the interstitium into the alveolar spaces.
e. The rapidity of blood flow precludes any transudation of fluid.

103   **In the normal person:**

a. The compliance of the combined lung–thorax (L–T) system is double that of the lungs alone.
b. The compliance of the combined L–T system is about 100 ml per centimetre water pressure.
c. The compliance of the combined L–T system increases relative to that of the lungs alone at the extremes of lung volume.
d. The work of the respiratory muscles is confined to the phase of inspiration.
e. Surface tension accounts for just one-third of the elastic forces in the lungs.

104   **During normal nasal breathing:**

a. The tidal air is almost fully saturated with water vapour before it leaves the nasal passages.
b. The tidal air temperature does not reach body temperature before the air reaches the carina.
c. Removal of foreign particulate matter occurs predominantly by filtration.
d. Particles the size of red blood cells normally reach the alveoli.
e. Cigarette smoke particles are precipitated in the conduits and normally don't reach the alveoli.

105   **At high altitudes such as the top of Mount Everest:**

a. The percentage of oxygen is the same as that at sea level.
b. The water vapour pressure in the alveoli is the same as that in alveoli at sea level provided the body temperature remains at 37°C.
c. The alveolar pCO_2 will remain the same as at sea level.
d. The diffusing capacity of oxygen through the pulmonary capillary membrane decreases.
e. There is a tendency to an increase in lung volume.

106 The blood volume of the lungs:

    a. Is about 500–1000 ml in the standard adult person.
    b. Is received in its entirety from the right ventricle.
    c. Is about equally distributed between the pulmonary arteries, capillaries and veins.
    d. Can be markedly reduced during a Valsalva manoeuvre.
    e. Can be a useful 'reservoir' to compensate for systemic blood loss.

107 The following are functions normally performed by the pulmonary endothelium:

    a. Phase II biotransformation of xenobiotics.
    b. Conversion of angiotensinogen into angiotensin I.
    c. Inactivation of serotonin (5 OH tryptamine).
    d. Manufacture of mast cells.
    e. Storage of arachidonic acid.

108 Surfactant:

    a. Stands for 'surface active agent'.
    b. Is secreted by Type I alveolar epithelial cells.
    c. Chemically is a single substance.
    d. Begins to form in the alveoli of the fetus in the first trimester of pregnancy.
    e. Normally helps decrease the water-produced surface tension about 4- to 5-fold.

109 In the standard adult person, when assuming the supine position from the erect position:

    a. The functional residual capacity is diminished.
    b. The expiratory reserve volume is decreased in the healthy person.
    c. The expiratory reserve volume is increased in the person with chronic obstructive pulmonary disease (COPD).
    d. Oesophageal sphincter tone is decreased.
    e. Gastric emptying time is prolonged.

110 Passive hyperventilation of a patient with atmospheric air at thrice the person's normal minute volume for about 5 minutes will lead to:

    a. A rise in arterial pO_2 to about 20 kPa.
    b. A fall in plasma potassium.
    c. A rise in the P_{50} of haemoglobin.
    d. A fall in plasma standard bicarbonate.
    e. A rise in urinary pH.

111 The following are largely removed from blood during its passage through the lungs:

a. Adrenaline.
b. Bradykinin.
c. Histamine.
d. Serotonin.
e. Vasopressin.

Physiology of the liver

112 At rest the liver:

    a. Contains about 15% of the total blood volume of the body.
    b. Has a blood flow comparable with that of the kidneys.
    c. Has about the same resting oxygen consumption as the heart.
    d. Has a higher blood flow per unit mass of tissue than the brain.
    e. Accounts for a greater percentage of body weight in an infant compared with an adult.

113 The liver:

    a. Is a manufacturing site for erythropoietin.
    b. Stores vitamin D.
    c. Breaks down nitrous oxide.
    d. Excretes calcium.
    e. Forms urobilinogen.

114 The liver is the only site in the body that:

    a. Manufactures albumin.
    b. Produces heparin.
    c. Manufactures vitamin K.
    d. Can form ketone bodies.
    e. Does not require insulin to permit ingress of glucose into cells.

Physiology of the brain

115 The following are true with respect to the brain:

a. Its glial cells make up about about one-quarter of the brain's cell volume.

b. Its grey matter blood flow is about twice that of the white matter.

c. Its activity accounts for about 20% of total basal oxygen consumption.

d. 60% of its energy expenditure is for electrophysiological function.

e. Its sole energy substrate is glucose.

116 The function of the blood–brain barrier (BBB) is impaired:

a. By clinical concentrations of inhalational anaesthetic agents.

b. Following a period of acute hypertension.

c. As a result of a rise in plasma osmolarity.

d. From the effects of microwave radiations.

e. During magnetic resonance imaging of the brain.

117 The following are features common to cerebral neuronal necrosis and cerebral neuronal apoptosis:

a. Cellular swelling.

b. Mitochondrial swelling.

c. Local infiltration by inflammatory cells.

d. Condensation of nuclear chromatin.

e. An acidophilic cytoplasm.

118 The following provide protection to brain cells after ischaemic injury:

a. Hypothermia.

b. Hyperglycaemia.

c. Hypercapnia.

d. Hypertension.

e. Acidosis.

119 The cerebrospinal fluid:

a. Is produced by a process of active secretion.

b. Has about the same specific gravity as brain tissue.

c. Has about the same osmolarity as plasma.

d. Is replaced about 8–10 times per day.

e. Has a hydrostatic pressure of about 10 mmHg in the supine position.

120   During pregnancy:

    a. The increase in body weight is predominantly due to the mass
       of the fetus and amniotic fluid.
    b. The cardiac output increases progressively until near term.
    c. The minute volume increases by about 50%.
    d. Base metabolic rate (BMR) increases uniformly during the 40
       weeks of gestation.
    e. There is a progressive increase in blood volume.

121   In pregnancy:

    a. Gastric motility is usually enhanced.
    b. The rate of absorption of intramuscular injections is more rapid.
    c. Both hepatic and renal blood flow are increased.
    d. There is generally a higher free fraction of drugs in the plasma.
    e. There may be increased cholinesterase activity.

122   The following changes occur in the infant at birth:

    a. Doubling of the systemic vascular resistance.
    b. Fall in pulmonary artery pressure.
    c. Closure of ductus venosus.
    d. Rise in portal venous pressure.
    e. Fall in blood sugar.

123   In relation to body weight the following parameters in a neonate
      are about twice their value in a standard young adult:

    a. Blood volume.
    b. Minute ventilation.
    c. Functional residual capacity.
    d. Cardiac output.
    e. Basal oxygen consumption.

124   Compared with an adult, the neonate:

    a. Has a higher gastric pH.
    b. Has a less permeable blood–brain barrier.
    c. Has significantly more absorption of dietary nutrients in the
       large intestine.
    d. Absorbs drugs faster from the GI tract.
    e. Has less efficient rectal absorption of drugs.

125   The following conditions have an autosomal dominant
      inheritance:

    a. Malignant hyperpyrexia.
    b. Porphyria.
    c. Haemophilia A.
    d. Glucose-6-phosphate dehydrogenase deficiency.
    e. Presence of atypical butyrylcholinesterase.

126   In the case of malignant hyperpyrexia:

a. The relevant gene is on chromosome 19.
b. Children have a higher incidence than adults.
c. The incidence is higher with suxamethonium than with any other anaesthetic agent.
d. A rise in temperature is usually the earliest manifestation.
e. There is a respiratory acidosis with a compensatory metabolic alkalosis.

127   Porphyria:

a. Is always an inherited condition.
b. Is more common as attacks in females.
c. Is often relieved by smoking.
d. Can be precipitated by dieting.
e. Is sometimes associated with hyponatraemia.

128   In the case of dystrophia myotonica:

a. It has a sex-linked recessive inheritance.
b. It normally first presents in adolescence.
c. There is an increase in creatinine kinase levels.
d. It is worsened by Class I antiarrhythmic agents.
e. It is ameliorated by pregnancy.

129   The following are accurate prognostic indicators of paracetamol poisoning:

a. Prothrombin time.
b. Lactic acidosis.
c. Measurement of coagulation Factor V by means of conventional tests.
d. Determination of Factor VIII levels by means of conventional tests.
e. Plasma creatinine levels.

130   Aspirin overdosage can lead to:

a. Hypocoagulability of blood.
b. Pulmonary oedema.
c. Hyperpyrexia.
d. Inappropriate ADH secretion.
e. Early loss of consciousness.

131　In constrictive pericarditis:

　　a. Patients may be vasoconstricted.
　　b. The jugular venous pressure falls during inspiration.
　　c. The jugular venous pressure graph is M-shaped due to exaggerated X and Y descent.
　　d. There is a visible expansile V-wave.
　　e. A third heart sound is usually present.

132　In Down's syndrome:

　　a. Atlanto-occipital instability is usually asymptomatic.
　　b. Cervical x-ray features are a reliable guide to atlanto-axial instability.
　　c. Thyroid hyperfunction is a common associated feature.
　　d. Ocular defects are relatively rare.
　　e. Cardiac defects are the commonest cause of mortality in infancy.

133　In the case of myasthenia gravis:

　　a. It is an antibody-mediated presynaptic disorder of the neuromuscular junction.
　　b. It can present right across the spectrum of life.
　　c. It presents more commonly with ocular features in oriental races.
　　d. The primary abnormality is loss of ACh receptors.
　　e. About three-quarters of patients show IgG antibodies.

134　In the case of the Eaton–Lambert (myasthenic) syndrome:

　　a. It is regarded as having an autoimmune aetiology.
　　b. The muscle weakness results from an abnormality at postsynaptic level.
　　c. Ocular muscle involvement is a standard feature.
　　d. When associated with malignancy it always follows the appearance of the tumour.
　　e. Autonomic dysfunction is a rare phenomenon.

135　In the case of OSA (obstructive sleep apnoea):

　　a. A narrow floppy upper airway is the site of pathophysiology.
　　b. Its origin may be congenital.
　　c. The condition is more pronounced during REM sleep.
　　d. There is pharyngeal collapse from the Bernoulli phenomenon.
　　e. The sufferer is invariably aware of the resulting sleep interruption.

136   **Failure of relaxation of the jaw following suxamethonium:**

a. Occurs as a normal response in c. 1% of the population.
b. Has been attributed to a variation in the structure of myosin.
c. May be the first sign of malignant hyperpyrexia.
d. May occur in patients with myotonia congenita.
e. Is not necessarily accompanied by peripheral muscle rigidity.

137   **The oculo-cardiac reflex:**

a. Has the trigeminal nerve as its afferent pathway.
b. Is more commonly activated during general anaesthesia in adults than in children.
c. Can when activated lead to ventricular fibrillation.
d. Can be activated during retrobulbar blockade.
e. Is fatigued, i.e. tends to be attenuated with repeated traction on ocular muscles.

138   **With increasing age:**

a. Total body water as a percentage of body mass is increased.
b. Lung compliance is decreased.
c. Serum creatinine rises.
d. The minimum alveolar concentration (MAC) requirement of inhalational anaesthetic agents falls.
e. The pH of gastric juice tends to rise.

Pharmacology

139   In the case of Phase I biotransformations:

a. They are solely dependent on the CYP 450 multifunction oxidase system.
b. They are exclusively localised in the endoplasmic reticulum.
c. They are essentially conjugation reactions.
d. They are the only form of reactions involved in leukotriene synthesis.
e. Their primary purpose is to render the xenobiotic agent easily excretable.

140   Conjugation in respect of drug biotransformation:

a. Is a Phase I process.
b. Is essentially a process that occurs in the endoplasmic reticulum.
c. Usually is a cytochrome P 450 oxidase function.
d. Has the effect of imparting hydrophobicity to the drug.
e. Can lead to the production of active metabolites.

141   Glucuronidation:

a. Is a Phase I biotransformation reaction:
b. Is a 'functionalisation' process.
c. Takes place in the cytosol.
d. Involves enzymes of the CYP 450 system.
e. In the case of morphine, can lead to the production of an active metabolite.

142   Drugs are more likely to be water soluble:

a. When they are in the form of a glucuronide conjugate.
b. When they have acquired a hydrocarbon chain.
c. On attachment of a steroid nucleus.
d. In the presence of a sulphate radical.
e. On acetylation.

143   Enzyme induction in relation to drugs:

a. Results from enhanced gene transcription.
b. Is an attribute predominantly of lipophilic drugs.
c. Can be due to a decreased rate of enzymatic degradation of the agent.
d. Has a direct relationship to the drugs' pharmacological properties.
e. Can even occur with inhalational anaesthetic agents.

144   Cytochrome oxidase P 450:

a. Is a haem-containing protein complex.
b. Is labelled '450' because of its maximum electronic magnetic radiations (EMR) absorption at a wavelength of 450 nm when coupled with carbon dioxide.
c. Is found in the rough endoplasmic reticulum.
d. Is a polyoxygenase system.
e. Is a mixed-function oxygenase system.

145   The following agents are structurally imidazoles:

a. Propofol.
b. Histamine.
c. Ketamine.
d. Etomidate.
e. Vasopressin.

146   The following statements are true:

a. Morphine is both an opiate and an opioid.
b. Thiopentone sodium is both a pyrimidine and a malonyl urea.
c. Vecuronium is both a steroid and a quaternary ammonium compound.
d. Atropine is both an acid and an amine.
e. Diclofenac is both an aniline and an acid.

147   The following have a plasma half-life measured in minutes:

a. Adenosine.
b. Adrenaline.
c. Antidiuretic hormone.
d. Insulin.
e. Nitric oxide.

148   Calcium:

a. Is actively absorbed in the proximal duodenum.
b. In its ionised form in the plasma accounts for only 50% of the plasma calcium content.
c. In its ionised form has an inverse relationship with the plasma parathyroid hormone level.
d. Is lowered in its plasma concentration by calcitonin.
e. Is required to bind with troponin to activate the actin–myosin interaction prior to muscle contraction.

149 **Angiotensin II:**

a. Is a directly acting vasoconstrictor.
b. Enhances the pre-junctional release of noradrenaline.
c. Increases ADH secretion by the posterior pituitary.
d. Stimulates aldosterone release from the adrenal cortex.
e. Degrades bradykinin.

150 **Xenon (in its role as an anaesthetic agent):**

a. Has a MAC value higher than N_2O.
b. Is a useful agent in patients with chronic obstructive pulmonary disease.
c. Has a higher blood gas partition coefficient than desflurane.
d. Has significant vasodilator properties.
e. Is not known to trigger malignant hyperpyrexia in susceptible swine.

151 **In the case of the barbiturates:**

a. They produce their effects by synaptic inhibition at $GABA_B$ receptors.
b. They cause a dose-dependent reduction in cerebral blood flow (CBF).
c. They cause a dose-dependent reduction in cerebral metabolic rate (CMR).
d. They reduce both electrical brain activity and cellular homeostasis in roughly equal measure.
e. Subjects may develop tolerance to them rapidly.

152 **Propofol:**

a. Is an alkyl phenol.
b. Is a chiral agent.
c. Is insoluble in water.
d. In its formulation for anaesthesia has a pH near that of plasma.
e. Is compatible with 5% glucose in water.

153 **The following are recognised additives in current preparations of propofol:**

a. Cremophor EL.
b. Sodium metabisulphite.
c. Soya bean oil.
d. Glycerol.
e. Benzethonium chloride.

154   Propofol is:

a. Hypnotic.
b. Sedative.
c. Anti-analgesic.
d. Anti-emetic.
e. Anti-epileptic.

155   The following IV induction agents produce their effects primarily by action at GABA receptors:

a. Thiopentone sodium.
b. Methohexitone.
c. Propofol.
d. Ketamine.
e. Etomidate.

156   Thiopentone sodium:

a. Is a pyrimidine derivative.
b. Is a substituted malonylurea.
c. Is presented as a tautomer.
d. Can be constituted with Hartmann's solution.
e. Owes its hypnotic effect to the parent barbiturate structure.

157   Ketamine:

a. Is almost devoid of hypnotic properties.
b. Is not safe for use in asthmatics.
c. Increases cerebral blood flow.
d. Relaxes jaw muscles almost as well as propofol.
e. Has β-adrenergic agonist actions.

158   Compared with ketamine, propofol:

a. Is a better analgesic.
b. Gives better relaxation of laryngeal and pharyngeal muscles.
c. Produces deeper anaesthesia.
d. Causes a higher level of tachycardia.
e. Produces no active metabolites.

159   Unpleasant emergence reactions after ketamine anaesthesia are more common:

a. In children compared with adults.
b. Women compared with men.
c. With concurrent administration of benzodiazepines.
d. With concurrently administered opioid analgesics.
e. Following concurrently administered nitrous oxide.

160 In the case of the inhalational anaesthetic agents halothane, enflurane, isoflurane, sevoflurane and desflurane:

a. They are all halogenated ethers.
b. They are all chiral agents.
c. They all contain preservatives in their manufactured form for anaesthetic use.
d. They are all amenable to measurement by ultraviolet analysis.
e. They can all be used safely with a low-flow breathing attachment with provision for CO_2 absorption with soda lime.

161 Epileptogenesis is a clinical concern with the following inhalational anaesthetic agents:

a. Halothane.
b. Enflurane.
c. Isoflurane.
d. Sevoflurane.
e. Desflurane.

162 The following are higher for desflurane compared with halothane, enflurane, isoflurane and sevoflurane:

a. Molecular weight.
b. Tendency to form carbon monoxide with soda lime.
c. Vapour pressure at room temperature.
d. MAC.
e. Biotransformation.

163 Halothane is the only halogenated inhalational anaesthetic agent:

a. That contains bromine.
b. That tarnishes metals.
c. That produces BCDFE with soda lime.
d. That does not have a CHF_2 moiety
e. That is reputed to cause an immunogenic hepatitis.

164 In the case of local anaesthetic agents:

a. Their lipophilicity is a property of their aromatic acid moiety.
b. Their degree of ionisation is dependent on their benzoic acid fraction.
c. Their potency is determined by their amino acid radical.
d. Their receptor affinity is an attribute of their benzoic acid moiety.
e. Their laevorotatory 'S' forms are usually more toxic than their dextrorotatory 'R' forms.

165 **Local anaesthetics:**

    a. Structurally are generally weak bases.
    b. Can exist in chiral forms.
    c. Are usually provided for clinical use as mildly acidic hydrochloride salts.
    d. Generally possess intrinsic vasodilator properties.
    e. Are bound in significant amounts on first pass to lung tissue.

166 **The following are generally true of local anaesthetic agents:**

    a. The ester LAs have a shorter plasma half-life.
    b. The amide LAs are more allergenic.
    c. S-enantiomers are better vasoconstrictors.
    d. R-enantiomers are more cardiotoxic.
    e. The amide LAs are not significantly bound to plasma proteins.

167 **The following local anaesthetic agents are both amide compounds and chiral agents:**

    a. Amethocaine.
    b. Bupivacaine.
    c. Lidocaine (lignocaine).
    d. Prilocaine.
    e. Ropivacaine.

168 **Cocaine:**

    a. Is obtained from *Chondrodendron tomentosum*.
    b. Is the only naturally occurring local anaesthetic.
    c. Prevents neuronal re-uptake of catecholamines.
    d. Inhibits monoamine oxidase.
    e. Is the only currently used LA with vasoconstricting activity.

169 **Lignocaine:**

    a. Is an aminoethyl amide.
    b. Can be used in patients allergic to ester type LAs.
    c. Is biotransformed by the mixed-function oxidase system of the liver.
    d. Produces metabolites which also have local anaesthetic activity.
    e. Produces metabolites that are voided from the body directly following biliary secretion.

170 Compared with lignocaine, bupivacaine:

a. Has a duration of action 2–3 times longer.
b. Has a toxicity 2–3 times greater.
c. Is many times more potent in blocking cardiac conduction.
d. Is better able to provide differential (i.e. sensory > motor) block.
e. Produces its cardiac effect partly by a central medullary action.

171 Prilocaine:

a. Is the least toxic of the amino amide LAs.
b. Undergoes metabolism in the liver, kidney *and* lung.
c. Causes more vasodilatation than most other LAs.
d. Is the only LA with potential to cause methaemoglobinaemia.
e. Is suitable for IV blockade because its increased 'volume of distribution' reduces its central nervous system (CNS) toxicity.

172 The following are now recognised as opioid receptor subtypes:

a. Mu (MOP).
b. Kappa (KOP).
c. Delta (DOP).
d. Sigma.
e. NOP (nociceptin orphanin FQ peptide).

173 Opioid receptor activation leads to:

a. Closing of voltage-sensitive Ca channels (VSCC).
b. Stimulation of K^+ efflux.
c. Inhibition of adenylyl cyclase.
d. Increased production of cAMP.
e. Activation of neurotransmitter release.

174 Mu opioid receptor activation:

a. Is the basis of pruritus.
b. Is the mechanism of opioid diuresis.
c. Is the causation of respiratory depression.
d. Leads to release of acetylcholine.
e. Is blocked by naloxone.

175 **Morphine:**

a. Is a benzylisoquinoline derivative.
b. Is highly selective for μ receptors.
c. Is a good analgesic for neuropathic pain.
d. Crosses the blood–brain barrier better than most other lipid-soluble opioids.
e. Produces a metabolite that has an even more potent analgesic effect.

176 **The respiratory depression of opioid analgesics:**

a. Is mediated through μ_2 receptors.
b. Is subject to a 'ceiling effect'.
c. Is usually accompanied by a reduction in both tidal volume and ventilation rate.
d. Is counteracted by hypoxia.
e. When reversed with naloxone involves some reversal of analgesia.

177 **Pethidine:**

a. Is a synthetic opioid analgesic.
b. Is a piperidine derivative.
c. Has a higher oral–parenteral potency ratio than morphine.
d. Readily crosses the placental barrier.
e. Shows a higher renal excretion on alkaline diuresis.

178 **Nalbuphine:**

a. Is a pure opioid agonist.
b. Is structurally related to naloxone.
c. Mediates its agonist actions at μ opioid receptors.
d. Is equianalgesic with morphine.
e. Is more prone to dysphoric effects than pentazocine.

179 **Propoxyphene:**

a. Is structurally related to methadone.
b. Is essentially a μ opioid agonist.
c. Possesses analgesic properties in all its stereo-isomers.
d. As an analgesic is as potent as oral codeine.
e. Is regarded as owing its toxicity to a metabolite.

180   Benzodiazepines:

a. Mediate their actions via $GABA_B$ receptors.
b. Are generally well bound to plasma proteins.
c. Are potent hepatic enzyme inducers.
d. Usually provide a dose-related protective effect against cerebral hypoxia.
e. Possess a potent anti-emetic effect.

181   Heparin:

a. Is a positively charged glycosaminoglycan.
b. Is released by basophils in the peripheral blood.
c. Is a potent anticoagulant in its own right.
d. Cannot be detected in the plasma under normal circumstances.
e. Is reversed by protamine by the process of pharmacological competitive antagonism.

182   Warfarin:

a. Is a racemic mixture in its clinically available preparation.
b. Is effective in vitro.
c. Is highly bound to plasma globulin.
d. Acts by a process of 'physiological' antagonism.
e. Is metabolised mainly in the liver.

183   The following are naturally occurring anticoagulants:

a. Glycocalyx.
b. Thrombomodulin.
c. Protein C.
d. α_2-macroglobulin.
e. Plasminogen.

184   Insulin:

a. Is a disulphide-linked polypeptide.
b. Has a molecular weight greater than that of albumin.
c. Is carried in the plasma bound to gamma globulin.
d. Increases urea production.
e. Increases the glucosyl valine adduct of haemoglobin A1c.

185   The following promote the secretion of insulin by the pancreas:

a. Glucose.
b. Amino acids.
c. Fatty acids.
d. Ketone bodies.
e. Somatostatin.

186   The following are biguanide antidiabetic agents:

a. Tolbutamide.
b. Chlorpropamide.
c. Glypizide.
d. Metformin.
e. Ciglitazone.

187   Metformin normalises blood sugar by the following mechanisms:

a. Increasing insulin release from the pancreas.
b. Increasing peripheral utilisation of glucose.
c. Inhibiting gluconeogenesis.
d. Reducing intestinal absorption of glucose.
e. Depressing glucagon secretion by the pancreas.

188   Nicotinic acetylcholine receptors (nAChRs) are found at the following sites:

a. Central nervous system.
b. Adrenal medulla.
c. Sympathetic ganglia.
d. Parasympathetic ganglia.
e. Sweat glands.

189   In the case of acetylcholinesterase:

a. It is an A type carboxylesterase.
b. It is present in its asymmetric form at neuromuscular junctions.
c. It is its esteratic site, not its anionic site, that is responsible for hydrolysing acetylcholine.
d. It undergoes carboxylation when acted on by anticholinesterases.
e. Its inactivation by anticholinesterases involves the formation of covalent bonds.

190   Magnetic nerve stimulation, as a means of monitoring neuromuscular block, has the following advantages over electrical stimulation:

a. It is less painful.
b. It does not require physical contact of stimulator with patient.
c. It is more accurate for Train-of-Four (TOF).
d. It can more easily provide for supramaximal stimulation.
e. The apparatus is even more portable.

191 The following are essential prerequisites of a peripheral nerve stimulator to elicit the degree of neuromuscular block:

a. The current must be a DC current.
b. The stimulus must have a sine wave configuration.
c. The wave must have a bi-phasic form.
d. The stimulus current ought not to be more than 80 mA.
e. The duration of the current must be between 0.5 and 1.0 ms.

192 In the case of depolarising neuromuscular block:

a. The TOF ratio is maintained.
b. Twitch height on TOF stimulation shows a reduction.
c. Peak muscle tension is sustained for the 5-second duration of tetanic stimulation.
d. Post-tetanic potentiation is a distinct possibility.
e. Anticholinesterases will reduce the degree of block.

193 Suxamethonium:

a. Acts at nicotinic receptor sites as well as muscarinic receptor sites.
b. Acts at both sympathetic and parasympathetic ganglia.
c. Can produce a bradycardia as well as a tachycardia.
d. Can induce hyperkalaemia as well as hypokalaemia.
e. Can cause a depolarising block as well as a non-depolarising block.

194 Adenosine:

a. Is an endogenous nucleotide.
b. Brings about its effects through G protein-coupled receptors.
c. Has a half-life of the order of a few minutes.
d. Is known to sensitise nociceptors.
e. Undergoes inactivation in the plasma by plasma esterases.

195 Postoperative nausea and vomiting (PONV) has a higher incidence in:

a. Children compared with adults.
b. Women rather than men.
c. The obese compared with the non-obese.
d. Prolonged pre-operative fasting rather than conventional pre-operative fasting.
e. Smokers than in non-smokers.

196 Metoclopramide:

a. Belongs to the class of benzamides.
b. Is structurally related to procainamide.
c. Readily crosses the placenta.
d. Has 5 HT_3 receptor antagonism.
e. Is excreted unchanged in the urine.

197 The following anti-emetics have been known to cause QT prolongation on the ECG:

a. Prochlorperazine.
b. Droperidol.
c. Metoclopramide.
d. Dexamethasone.
e. Cyclizine.

198 In the case of each of the following drugs, one enantiomer has a pharmacological effect entirely different from the usual (and desired) effect of the other enantiomer:

a. Halothane.
b. Ketamine.
c. Propranolol.
d. Thalidomide.
e. Verapamil.

199 Aspirin:

a. Is an ester of salicylic acid.
b. Is a pro-drug.
c. Is only slightly bound to plasma proteins.
d. Is normally renally excreted unchanged.
e. On long-term used is reputed to lead to addiction.

200 Aspirin is best avoided in:

a. Children.
b. Asthmatics.
c. Porphyria.
d. Glucose-6-phosphate dehydrogenase deficiency.
e. Colonic polyposis.

201 When present in the following, aspirin is more likely to be found in a greater percentage in the ionised form than the unionised form:

a. Gastric lumen.
b. Gastric epithelial cell.
c. Lower small intestinal lumen.
d. Plasma.
e. Urine of pH about 6.5.

202 Paracetamol:

a. Is a chiral drug.
b. Is an active metabolite of phenacetin.
c. Has analgesic, antipyretic and anti-inflammatory properties.
d. Has no cyclooxygenase inhibitory effects whatsoever.
e. Is largely eliminated unchanged in the urine.

203 The following analgesics are best avoided during warfarin treatment:

a. Aspirin.
b. Paracetamol.
c. Diclofenac.
d. Dextropropoxyphene.
e. Ketorolac.

204 The following drugs tend to cause methaemoglobinaemia:

a. Prilocaine.
b. Aspirin.
c. Primaquine.
d. Phenacetin.
e. Dapsone.

205   The following are non-dimensional quantities, i.e. they are mere ratios, percentages or fractions and have no attached units:

a. Therapeutic index.
b. Cardiac index.
c. Quetelet index.
d. Substitution index.
e. Relative refractive index.

206   The following are non-dimensional quantities, i.e. they are mere ratios, percentages or fractions and have no attached units:

a. Hill coefficient.
b. Faraday constant.
c. Reynolds' number.
d. Reflection coefficient.
e. Dielectric constant.

207   The following are calculated, and not measured, parameters:

a. Clearance.
b. Volume of distribution of an agent.
c. Standard bicarbonate.
d. Free water.
e. Resting lung volume.

208   The following physical units express 'intensity' or 'concentration', i.e. a quantity per unit surface area:

a. Ampere.
b. Lumen.
c. Pascal.
d. Watt.
e. Weber.

209   The following are approximate equivalents of 1 atmosphere pressure:

a. 760 torr.
b. 1000 centimetres water.
c. 1,000,000 newtons per square metre.
d. 100,000 dynes per square centimetre.
e. 14 pounds per square inch.

210 The following are temperature dependent:

a. Osmolarity of a solution.
b. Mass of a substance.
c. Blood-gas partition coefficient.
d. Ostwald solubility coefficient.
e. Speed of light in a vacuum.

211 The following relationships when graphically represented take the form of a rectangular hyperbola:

a. The variation of pressure with volume of a fixed mass of gas at constant temperature.
b. The electrical capacitance of a capacitor and the distance between the capacitor plates.
c. The stimulus strength and the stimulus duration required for depolarisation of a membrane.
d. The viscosity of blood and its haematocrit.
e. The rate of elimination of an agent in accordance with zero-order kinetics.

212 The definition of an 'ideal gas' entails the following:

a. The gas molecules are regarded as 'dimensionless entities'.
b. The intermolecular collisions are perfectly elastic.
c. Collisions between the molecules and the container walls are perfectly elastic.
d. The gas must have a critical temperature below 273 K.
e. Van der Waals' forces ought to exist between molecules.

213 The following are definitional attributes of an 'ideal fluid':

a. The fluid is incompressible.
b. The flow of the fluid conforms to the Hagen–Poiseuille law.
c. The fluid is thixotropic.
d. The fluid has a dynamic viscosity the same as its kinematic viscosity.
e. The fluid has a density that remains constant despite changes in flow rate.

214 The following are attributes of laser light:

a. Collimation.
b. Coherence.
c. Cavitation.
d. Precession.
e. Population inversion.

215 The following are components that determine the dynamic response of an invasive arterial blood pressure monitoring transducer:

a. Mass of moving parts.
b. Stiffness of system.
c. Viscous drag in fluid column.
d. Velocity of fluid movement in tubing.
e. Natural resonant frequency of the transducer system.

216 Oxygen cylinders:

a. When full have a gauge pressure of approximately 137 bar, no matter the size of cylinder.
b. Can safely be made of aluminium.
c. Have a black body and black and white shoulders.
d. Have a filling ratio of 0.75 in temperate countries.
e. Have the pin index positions 3 and 5.

217 The following are correct pin index positions:

a. Nitrous oxide: 3 and 5.
b. Air: 1 and 6.
c. Carbon dioxide: 1 and 5.
d. Entonox: 7.
e. Cyclopropane: 3 and 6.

218 The following statements are true:

a. A size F oxygen cylinder cannot be attached to a present-day anaesthetic machine solely for reasons of cylinder height.
b. A size E carbon dioxide cylinder cannot be coupled to an anaesthetic machine (which has pin index provision for CO_2 flow).
c. If cyclopropane is to be provided from cylinders on an anaesthetic machine, a pressure regulator is essential in the gas pathway.
d. The pressure regulators for the oxygen and nitrous oxide pathways on an anaesthetic machine are freely interchangeable.
e. Pipeline air to an anaesthetic machine is provided at the same pressure as the pipeline air for surgical drills.

219 Oxygen can be measured by the following methods:

a. Mass spectrometry.
b. Infra-red analysis.
c. Raman scattering.
d. Paramagnetic analysis.
e. Pyrogallol method.

220 Of the methods available for gas analysis:

a. Infra-red analysis can be used to measure N_2O.
b. Raman scattering can measure helium.
c. The piezo-electric method is suitable for estimating sevoflurane.
d. Halothane can be assayed by the method of ultraviolet analysis.
e. Mass spectrometry can be used to measure all the agents mentioned in a through d above.

221 In the case of the 'Clark electrode' method for measurement of oxygen:

a. The device requires an 'external' source of energy.
b. The two electrodes can be of the same material.
c. The definitive reaction (i.e. that which enables determination of the O_2 tension) occurs at the anode.
d. The definitive reaction is analogous to that produced by O_2 in the Krebs tricarboxylic cycle.
e. Its performance is unaffected by temperature change.

222 In the case of anaesthetic breathing attachments:

a. The Waters' to-and-fro attachment is a Mapleson A attachment.
b. The Bain co-axial attachment is more efficient than the Magill in spontaneous ventilation mode.
c. The Lack attachment has an inner co-axial afferent limb.
d. The Ayre's T-piece breathing attachment suitably upsized can be used for adult spontaneous ventilation.
e. The Magill attachment suitably downsized can be used effectively in the spontaneous ventilation mode for infants.

223 When an adult person is undergoing spontaneous ventilation with a fresh gas flow rate sufficient to maintain normocapnia, the 'breathing' bag in each of the following contains essentially fresh gases:

a. Magill attachment.
b. Bain co-axial attachment.
c. Lack co-axial attachment.
d. Parallel Lack attachment.
e. Waters' to-and-fro breathing attachment as used in recovery wards.

224 Compared with a Magill anaesthetic breathing attachment, the following attachments are more 'efficient' for spontaneous ventilation:

a. A Bain co-axial attachment.
b. A Waters' to-and-fro attachment.
c. A Lack co-axial attachment.
d. A parallel Lack attachment.
e. An Ayres T-piece attachment with Jackson Rees modification.

225 Water is regarded as an essential pre-requisite in soda lime preparations because:

a. The chemical reactions involved in CO_2 absorption will not take place in its absence.
b. Its absence will predispose to greater carbon monoxide production.
c. Wetness of the soda lime will improve CO_2 absorption by the granules.
d. Its presence will significantly improve humidification of inspired gases.
e. Its absence will markedly increase the formation of Compound A with sevoflurane.

226 During low-flow anaesthesia when using a circle breathing attachment (with provision for CO_2 absorption) the following contaminants have been known to accumulate as a result of reaction between soda lime and inhalational agents:

a. Carbonyl chloride.
b. Methane.
c. Nitrogen dioxide.
d. Trifluoromethylvinyl ether.
e. Bromochlorodifluoroethylene.

227 The 'pumping effect' in respect of plenum vaporisers is less marked if:

a. There is a long tortuous inlet tube into the vaporising chamber.
b. The bi-metallic strip is placed in the vaporising chamber rather than the bypass chamber.
c. There is a non-return valve just downstream of the exit port of the vaporiser.
d. There is a non-return valve just upstream of the inlet port of the vaporiser.
e. The vaporising chamber has less liquid anaesthetic agent rather than more.

228 The following are or have been used as plenum vaporisers:

a. Boyle bottle.
b. Goldman vaporiser.
c. EMO (Epstein Macintosh Oxford) vaporiser.
d. Desflurane vaporiser.
e. TEC Mark 4 Penlon PPV vaporiser.

229 The conventional TEC Mark 4 plenum isoflurane vaporiser is a:

a. Variable-bypass vaporiser.
b. Flow over vaporiser.
c. Temperature compensated vaporiser.
d. Out-of-breathing-circuit vaporiser.
e. Concentration-calibrated vaporiser.

230 The 'TEC Mark 6' desflurane vaporiser:

a. Is a plenum vaporiser.
b. Works on the 'splitting ratio' principle.
c. Needs to be energised by electricity for its proper functioning.
d. Produces vapour at a partial pressure of c. 200 kPa at sea level.
e. Delivers a constant partial pressure of the agent vapour, no matter the ambient pressure.

231 In the present-day anaesthetic machine, oxygen at a pressure of 400 kPa:

a. Flows up the oxygen flowmeter tube.
b. Operates the oxygen cut-off warning device.
c. Feeds the oxygen flush.
d. Provides the driving energy for the Manley MP 3 ventilator.
e. Can be used satisfactorily to inflate a Hg sphygmomanometer cuff.

232 The gas flow tubes of a flowmeter unit of the present-day anaesthetic machine:

a. Work on the 'variable orifice/constant pressure differential' principle.
b. Need not be rendered antistatic, now that no flammable anaesthetic agents are in use.
c. Need to be inclined slightly from the vertical for their proper functioning.
d. Are influenced in their flow rates by *both* the density and the viscosity of the gases.
e. Are non-interchangeable for reasons of height alone.

233   The following are true in respect of the oxygen flush control of
       the present-day anaesthetic machine:

a. It is supplied by oxygen at a pressure of 400 kPa.
b. It is mandatory that it provides oxygen at a flow rate of 30–40
   L/minute.
c. The regulations require that it shall not be lockable in the
   'ON' position.
d. When operational it must cut off the N_2O flow up the
   rotameter tube.
e. When operational it must necessarily cut off the flow of O_2 up
   the rotameter tube.

234   The following are essential for the proper performance of CO_2
       absorption by soda lime:

a. Moisture.
b. Sodium hydroxide.
c. Calcium hydroxide.
d. Potassium hydroxide.
e. Granularity.

235   Conductive gel is used in the following situations to reduce
       electrical impedance:

a. Electrodes when recording an ECG.
b. To attach defibrillator pads to the chest wall for the purpose
   of cardioconversion.
c. When applying a diathermy pad.
d. To connect the leads of a peripheral nerve stimulator for
   monitoring neuromuscular block.
e. When applying an ultrasound probe during an US investigation.

236   The usual operational frequency of the following appliances is
       in the megahertz range or higher:

a. Diathermy (electrosurgical) unit.
b. Ultrasound diagnostic machine.
c. Carbon dioxide laser.
d. 'Harmonic scalpel'.
e. The infra-red thermometer.

237   The use of DC electric current rather than AC current:

a. Eliminates the risk of electrocution by ventricular fibrillation.
b. Makes the production of a laser light beam impossible.
c. Is to all intents and purposes necessary for successful
   cardioconversion.
d. Will not allow the proper performance of ultrasound imaging.
e. Will negate any possibility of the use of electrical cautery.

238 **The following statements are correct with respect to electrical equipment:**

a. Class I equipment has a three-wire cable, one wire of which is the protective earth.
b. Class II equipment has no designated symbol.
c. Class III equipment is 'internally powered'.
d. A properly working 'protective earth' on an appliance will keep the equipment casing at near-zero potential.
e. The permitted 'leakage current' for CF-type electrical equipment must be less than that for BF-type equipment.

239 **The following statements are true with respect to electricity:**

a. In an AC circuit the current never reaches steady-state conditions.
b. The current 'through' a capacitor is proportional to the rate of change of applied voltage.
c. The higher the frequency of alternation of an AC current the lower the reactance in an inductor in the circuit.
d. The opposition to current flow in an AC circuit containing a capacitor and an inductor is measured in mhos.
e. A DC circuit containing solely a resistor will have resistance but no reactance.

240 **The use of an 'REM' return electrode monitoring diathermy plate:**

a. Is only possible with an 'isolated' diathermy unit.
b. Markedly reduces the likelihood of a skin burn under the diathermy plate.
c. Is essential for use of the 'cutting' mode.
d. Is unnecessary if bipolar diathermy is being used.
e. Is essential if the diathermy switch is being hand operated.

241 **Oxygen:**

a. Is a paramagnetic gas.
b. Possesses two unpaired electrons in each atom.
c. Absorbs ultraviolet light.
d. Can be measured by mass spectrometry.
e. Is an ideal 'electron sink' for the energy-generating electron transport system.

242 **Nitrogen:**

a. Is a paramagnetic gas.
b. Is a narcotic at high pressures.
c. Has a higher solubility coefficient than oxygen in plasma.
d. Is less soluble in body fat than in body water.
e. Is present in the human body in a greater volume as gaseous nitrogen than as dissolved nitrogen.

243 In the case of carbon dioxide:

a. It constitutes about 0.3% of atmospheric air.
b. In cylinder form can be attached to the anaesthetic machine as C, D or E cylinder sizes.
c. In a full cylinder it is present at the same pressure as a full oxygen cylinder.
d. When combining with soda lime it does so as an endothermic reaction.
e. It is enzyme dependent for its combination with haemoglobin to form carbaminohaemoglobin.

244 Concerning helium:

a. Its viscosity is lower than that of nitrogen.
b. It has the lowest density of all gases.
c. Is of use in lower airway obstruction.
d. It can be estimated by Raman scattering.
e. It is the only gas that still remains in liquid form at near-zero kelvin.

245 Nitrous oxide:

a. Is obtained for anaesthetic use from natural gas.
b. In solution is sweeter than sucrose.
c. Is a vigorous supporter of combustion.
d. Produces its anaesthetic effect by acting on GABA receptors.
e. Is excreted from the body solely by exhalation via the lungs.

246 If a nitrous oxide cylinder on an anaesthetic machine is 'bled' at a constant and rapid rate:

a. The pressure gauge will show a linear change with time.
b. The outside of the cylinder can become frosted.
c. The amount of nitrous oxide remaining in the cylinder can be determined correctly only by weighing the cylinder.
d. The cylinder can stop releasing its gas if water were a contaminant of its contents.
e. There is a risk of other oxides of nitrogen forming inside the cylinder.

247 The reading on the pressure gauge on the following cylinders accurately reflects the amount of gas in them:

a. Oxygen.
b. Nitrous oxide.
c. Helium.
d. Carbon dioxide.
e. Entonox.

248   **The thermistor (as a method of temperature measurement):**

    a. Is based on the activity of semi-conductor materials.
    b. Has a 'positive temperature coefficient'.
    c. Measures voltage changes with varying temperature.
    d. Is very sensitive to small changes in temperature.
    e. Tends to show hysteresis.

Materia miscellanea

249   Hydrogen bonds:

    a. Are weaker than covalent bonds.
    b. Are present in water.
    c. Contribute to the globular shape of proteins.
    d. Help stabilise the double helix of DNA.
    e. Are integral bonds in the structure of methane.

250   van der Waals' interactions:

    a. Are strong intramolecular forces.
    b. Are bonding attractions.
    c. Account for the non-ideal behaviour gases.
    d. Explain the lattice energy of molecular crystals.
    e. Obey the Inverse Square Law with respect to the relationship between the product of the magnitude of the forces and the distance separating them.

251   The chemical reactions in the following involve linkage by means of covalent bonding:

    a. The reaction of $Ca(OH)_2$ in soda lime with CO_2 to form $CaCO_3$.
    b. The inactivation of cyclo-oxygenase by aspirin.
    c. The neutralisation of heparin by protamine sulphate.
    d. The chelation of calcium by edetate.
    e. The combination of CO_2 with the plasma proteins to form carbamate.

252   *cis-trans* isomerism:

    a. Is the same as geometric isomerism.
    b. Is a type of dynamic isomerism.
    c. Is only possible in the presence of chemical double bonds.
    d. Is a feature of fatty acids of the cell membrane.
    e. Has an essential role in vision.

253   Free radicals:

    a. Are species with an unpaired electron.
    b. Usually result from heterolytic fission of covalent bonds.
    c. In the case of oxygen can be 'diradical' in form.
    d. Plays a role in polymerisation reactions.
    e. As primary pollutants are released from vehicle exhaust emissions.

254 Superoxide formation:

a. Is the basis of phagocytic destruction of bacterial cells.
b. Is implicated in the genesis of arthritic damage.
c. Is regarded as a contributory factor in ageing.
d. Is said to contribute to cataract formation.
e. Is now said to be the pathological basis of heart attacks.

255 The following are biological quenching agents (i.e. antioxidants):

a. Alpha tocopherol.
b. Beta-carotene.
c. Gamma-aminobutyric acid.
d. Delta-aminolevulinic acid.
e. Epsilon-aminocaproic acid.

256 In the process of body heat loss by radiation:

a. The loss usually accounts for about 25% of total body heat loss.
b. The loss is in the form of emission of ultraviolet EMRs.
c. The heat loss can occur even if the body were in a vacuum.
d. The loss can occur even against a temperature gradient.
e. Other things being equal, the loss is greater in a fair-skinned compared with a dark-skinned person.

257 When acting as sterilants, aliphatic alcohols:

a. Act by denaturing bacterial proteins.
b. Are more bactericidal the longer their chain length.
c. Are more effective as isoforms than as unbranched ('straight-chain') alcohols.
d. Are more active the higher their concentration.
e. Are effective against both Gram-positive and Gram-negative organisms.

258 The following disinfectants are reputed to be sporicidal with conventional usage:

a. Alcohols.
b. Povidone iodine.
c. Chlorine compounds.
d. Formaldehyde.
e. Chlorhexidine.

259   The following statements are true:

a. Heparin is the strongest acid in the body.
b. Acetylcholine is the only endogenous agent that causes both hypotension and bradycardia.
c. Calcium is the only inorganic clotting factor.
d. Nitrous oxide is the only inhalational anaesthetic agent that does not undergo biotransformation.
e. Helium is the only gas that still remains liquid at a temperature near 0 K.

260   Under normal circumstances the following usually have a pressure that is slightly subatmospheric:

a. The intrapleural pressure during the whole respiratory cycle.
b. The subalveolar interstitial space.
c. Abdominal cavity.
d. Synovial space of joints.
e. Epidural space.

1 **Answers**

    a. False – remember the 'mantra': 'LR 6, SO 4, all the rest by 3': lateral rectus by the 6th (abducens), superior oblique by the 4th (trochlear), all the rest by the 3rd (oculomotor).

    b. True – its dorsal attachment is very small and may be absent.

    c. False – the vagus nerve gives a cutaneous supply to a small area just in front of the auricle.

    d. False – the basilar artery is also unpaired.

    e. False – the lumbar segments 1 and 2 also do. The intermediolateral horn is the site of sympathetic relay within the cord and therefore must be present in segments T1–L2.

2 **Answers**

    a. True – supplies most of the eye muscles and also conveys parasympathetic motor fibres to the ciliary muscle.

    b. True – supplies the lateral rectus muscle of the eye.

    c. False – the lingual nerve supplies the mucous membrane of the anterior two-thirds of the tongue. It has no motor component.

    d. False – the glossopharyngeal has several sensory components: (i) the tympanic branch, which has sensory branches from the middle ear and the auditory tube; (ii) the supply to the mucous membrane of the posterior third of the tongue; (iii) a pharyngeal branch to the wall of the pharynx; and (iv) a sinus branch to the carotid sinus and body.

    e. True – it is the motor supply to sternomastoid and trapezius muscles.

3 **Answers**

    a. True – about 75%.

    b. True – about 75–80% of vagal fibres are sensory.

    c. False – it is through the jugular foramen.

    d. False – through the oesophageal opening.

    e. False – only as far as the transverse colon.

4 **Answers**

    a. False – it extends from C3 to the lower border of C6.

    b. False – all except the cricothyroid, which is supplied by the external laryngeal nerve.

    c. False – except for that lining the vocal cords, which is stratified squamous.

    d. False – the recurrent laryngeal nerve supplies the mucosa below the vocal cords. The internal laryngeal nerve supplies above the cords.

    e. False – the superior thyroid artery supplies the upper half of the larynx; the inferior thyroid supplies the lower half.

5 **Answers**

a. **True** – for about 2.5 cm.
b. **False** – it is the 3rd thoracic vertebra.
c. **True**.
d. **False** – the 10th rib.
e. **True**.

6 **Answers**

a. **True**.
b. **False** – a small amount occurs directly into the ventricular cavities via small venae cordis minimae, the 'thebesian veins'.
c. **False** – the 3rd cranial nerve arises from the Edinger–Westphal nucleus in the midbrain.
d. **False** – the first cervical nerve has no cutaneous distribution.
e. **True**.

7 **Answers**

a. **True** – arises from the anterior roots of cervical nerves 3, 4 and 5.
b. **False** – the phrenic nerve also contains some sensory (proprioceptive) fibres for the diaphragm, as well as sensory fibres to the pleura and peritoneum covering the upper and lower surfaces of the central part of the diaphragm.
c. **True**.
d. **False** – descends on the anterior aspect of the scalenus anterior, moving across it from its lateral to its medial aspect.
e. **False** – the phrenic nerve enters the thorax in front of the subclavian artery and behind the brachiocephalic vein.

8 **Answers**

a. **True**.
b. **False** – Type C fibres are the small unmyelinated fibres that conduct impulses at low velocities and constitute more than one half of sensory fibres.
c. **True** – δ-type fibres are a subcategory of Type A fibres and also convey pricking pain sensations.
d. **True**.
e. **True**.

9   **Answers**

a. **False** – the right coronary artery arises from the anterior aortic sinus and the left from the left posterior aortic sinus.
b. **True**.
c. **True**.
d. **False** – the cardiac sympathetic supply is from the cervical and upper thoracic portions of the sympathetic trunks and therefore from the 1st four thoracic spinal segments.
e. **False** – the left vagus nerve supplies the atrioventricular node and the sinoatrial node is supplied by the right vagus nerve.

10   **Answers**

a. **False** – although about 75% of vagal fibres are sensory, the vagus nerves are regarded as being devoid of afferent pain fibres.
b. **False** – postganglionic sympathetic fibres are usually devoid of myelin sheaths.
c. **False** – sympathetic fibres to the sweat glands and piloerector muscles have acetylcholine as their transmitter substance, i.e. they are 'sympathetic' but 'cholinergic'.
d. **True** – in the case of the sympathetic fibres to the adrenal medulla.
e. **False** – the supply via the 3rd cranial nerve arises in the Edinger–Westphal nucleus in the midbrain (and innervates the ciliary muscle).

11   **Answers**

a. **False** – it is about 5–10 nm thick. (1 nm = 10 Å).
b. **False** – it is an 'amphipathic' structure, i.e. it possesses both hydrophobic and hydrophilic moieties. An amphoteric substance is one that acts as both an acid and a base, e.g. amino acids. (Water too is amphoteric because it can dissociate into OH^- and H^+ radicals).
c. **False** – it is asymmetric in structure due to the irregular distribution of proteins within the membrane and it also has an 'inside-outside' asymmetry because of the location of carbohydrates attached to membrane proteins.
d. **True** – the essence of the fluid mosaic model is that membranes are two-dimensional solutions of oriented lipids and globular proteins. The lipid layer has a dual role: to act both as a solvent for integral membrane proteins and as a permeability barrier.
e. **False** – a 'micelle' has only one lipid layer. The cell membrane resembles a 'liposome' in that it has two lipid layers with their hydrophobic ends facing each other.

12   Answers

a. **True** – because it creates an electrical gradient across the cell membrane.
b. **True**.
c. **True** – by keeping sodium out of cells it reduces the number of osmotically active intracellular particles and thereby prevents massive water ingress into cells.
d. **True**.
e. **True** – Digoxin inhibits the Na^+–K^+–ATPase pump. This leads to a higher level of Na^+ inside the cell, leading to a diminished extracellular/intracellular Na^+ gradient, which results in slower extrusion of Ca^{2+} by the Na^+/Ca^{2+} exchanger. The consequent increase in intracellular Ca^{2+} enhances contractility of the cardiac muscle.

13   Answers

a. **True** – bulk flow is the transmembranal flow of water through aqueous pores or between adjacent cells. (Note: water movement is always passive and is dependent on the presence of a hydrostatic or osmolar gradient).
b. **True** – it is the same as 'bulk flow', but refers to the 'drag' of solute by the solvent. When a solvent moves across a partition because of physical absorptive forces, movement of the solvent will 'drag' any solutes present by convection.
c. **True**.
d. **True** – it is a form of carrier-mediated transport, from high to low concentration, in which solute molecules bind to specific membrane protein carriers, which thereby 'facilitate' their journey through the membrane.
e. **False** – pinocytosis is one form of endocytosis – phagocytosis is another – and is a process of uptake by cells of small particles in the form of vesicles. The process requires ATP and possesses selectivity.

Note: in strict physical theory all movement, even simple diffusion, requires some energy. In 'passive' transport processes there is no requirement for 'external' energy, the 'momentum' for movement being provided by the 'intrinsic' energy of the molecules themselves.

14   Answers

a. **False** – it can also occur through cellular channels.
b. **False** – shows zero-order kinetics. In first-order kinetics a constant *fraction* of the solute diffuses per unit time. In zero order kinetics a constant *amount* of the solute diffuses per unit time.
c. **False**.
d. **False** – it is directly proportional to the concentration gradient: Fick's law of diffusion.
e. **False** – it is inversely proportional to the square root of the molecular weight: Graham's Law of diffusion: $D \propto \dfrac{1}{\sqrt{MW}}$

15 **Answers**

a. **True**.
b. **True**.
c. **False** – not always. Cellular energy is not required in the case of facilitated diffusion, which is one form of carrier-mediated transport.
d. **True** – as happens in primary active transport which is a carrier-mediated process.
e. **True** – because it depends on the carrier protein, which is present in finite amount and therefore can become 'saturated'.

16 **Answers**

a. **True**.
b. **False** – facilitated diffusion cannot occur against a concentration gradient.
c. **True** – once the carrier protein is 'saturated', the rate of transfer cannot keep pace with the substrate concentration.
d. **True** – because they depend on proteins, which are temperature sensitive. (In fact all forms of transmembranal transport, including passive diffusion, are affected by temperature, because a rise in temperature will increase the kinetic energy of the molecules and thus increase their activity and therefore their movement).
e. **False** – facilitated diffusion is utilised as a form of transmembranal transfer of glucose using glucose transporter (GLUT) 1–5. Glucose is not transported into cells by a primary active mechanism. However, it is transported by a secondary active process involving sodium viz. sodium-dependent glucose transporter (SGLT 1), which is a symporter.

17 **Answers**

a. **True**.
b. **True** – pleiotropy is the ability of a single extracellular signal to generate multiple responses in a target cell.
c. **True** – into a larger α subunit and a smaller β/γ subunit.
d. **False** – fast synaptic transmission between cells is the function of ion channels.
e. **False** – it is $GABA_A$ receptors that are responsible for the mode of action of most anaesthetic agents, an important exception being ketamine, which acts by antagonising glutamate at N-methyl-D-aspartate (NMDA) receptors.

18   Answers

a. False – AMPA receptors are ionotropic receptors.
b. True.
c. True.
d. True – they are in fact one subtype of glutamate receptors.
e. True.

Note: In ionotropic receptors the transmitter binding site and the transmembrane ion channel are integral to a single protein complex. Therefore binding of the transmitter directly and immediately alters the activity of the ion channel, and thus ionotropic receptors are fast transmitter channels, acting over a time scale of milliseconds, for example the nicotinic acetylcholine receptor of skeletal NMJ. In metabotropic receptors the transmitter receptor and the effector are two separate entities and therefore the time course of their activity is slower – seconds or sometimes even minutes, for example the β-adrenergic receptor of cardiomyocyte.

19   Answers

a. False – an amphibolic pathway is one that can proceed in both directions. The Krebs cycle is an amphibolic pathway.
b. False – it occurs in the cytosol.
c. False – although its presence is useful, oxygen is not essential for its reactions. In other words, oxygen is 'facultative', not 'obligatory', for the reaction.
d. False – CO_2 is not a product of its reactions.
e. False – it produces four molecules of ATP per molecule of glucose consumed. But since two ATP molecules are consumed in the process, the net production is only two, compared with the Krebs cycle, which produces 36 molecules of ATP.

20   Answers

a. True – an autacoid is a substance that produces its effect either on the very cell that releases it (autocrine effect) or on a cell very near it (paracrine effect): The word 'autacoid' comes from the Greek words *auto*, meaning 'self' and *acos*, meaning 'remedy'). By contrast, hormones produce an 'endocrine' effect because they act at locations far removed from their site of production.
b. True – abluminal side: the side opposite to the lumen, therefore the 'basement membrane' side.
c. False – it is true of nitric oxide, but prostaglandins act via adenylyl cyclase.
d. False – NO: duration of action: a few seconds; prostacyclin: duration of action: 2–3 minutes.
e. False – prostacyclin does but NO cannot because the release of NO by the endothelium is dependent on the vasodilatory action of acetylcholine at muscarinic receptors on the endothelium and the integrity of the latter is necessary for such release.

21 **Answers**

    a. True.
    b. True – due to its higher lipid content.
    c. True.
    d. False – gives a white colour because of its higher refractive index.
    e. False – most axons within the CNS do not have (myelin) sheaths.

22 **Answers**

    a. False – EDRF refers to NO produced by the endothelium alone (see also MCQ 36).
    b. True – is dependent on NO synthase, which converts arginine to citrulline in the process.
    c. True.
    d. True – acts by combining with the haem in guanylyl cyclase to produce its effects.
    e. False – the half-life of NO is of the order of a few seconds.

23 **Answers**

    a. True.
    b. False – causes pulmonary vasodilatation but not systemic vasodilatation because it is rapidly inactivated by haemoglobin.
    c. True – (see **b.**)
    d. True – in the process of being inactivated by haemoglobin the NO converts the ferrous iron into ferric and thus the haemoglobin to methaemoglobin.
    e. True – N_2O_4, which is then converted to nitrous and nitric acids.

24 **Answers**

    a. False – pre-ganglionic fibres are myelinated (and are white in colour); postganglionic fibres are non-myelinated (and are grey in colour).
    b. False – myelinated fibres have a higher lipid content, which gives them a higher refractive index and therefore a white appearance.
    c. False – they originate in the intermedio-lateral horns (of spinal segments T1–L2).
    d. False – it is the pre-ganglionic fibres.
    e. True – via the stellate ganglion and cervical ganglia.

25 Answers

a. **False** – pre-ganglionic fibres are much longer than postganglionic fibres because the ganglia are very near their target organs (cx. sympathetic fibres).

b. **False** – the 3rd cranial nerve outflow originates in the Edinger–Westphal nucleus in the midbrain; the outflows of the other nerves (VII, IX and X) originate in the medulla.

c. **True** – nearly 75%.

d. **True**.

e. **False** – the predominant supply is sympathetic.

26 Answers

a. **True**.

b. **False**.

c. **False**.

d. **False** – the ganglion impar is the sympathetic terminal (single) midline ganglion and is situated on the anterior aspect of the coccyx and therefore is also known as the coccygeal ganglion.

e. **False**.

27 Answers

a. **False** – the vagus and not the sympathetic nervous system is the predominant influence.

b. **True** – α_1-adrenergic agonism.

c. **False** – bronchomotor tone is essentially under vagal influence.

d. **False** – GI activity is predominantly under parasympathetic control.

e. **True** – α_1-adrenergic agonism.

28 Answers

a. **True** – α_1 agonism.

b. **True** – β_2 agonism.

c. **True** – α_1 agonism.

d. **True** – β_2 agonism.

e. **False** – sympathetic agonism leads to ADH release.

29 Answers

a. **True** – it is the choline that is the quaternary ammonium moiety.
b. **True** – it is also a nicotinic agonist because it is the transmitter at autonomic ganglia and the skeletal neuromuscular (NM) junction, as well as some postganglionic sympathetic sites, i.e. sweat glands and piloerector muscles.
c. **True** – indeed it is the only endogenous agent known to cause both hypotension and bradycardia.
d. **True** – thereby delays resumption of threshold potential and thus the ability to generate another action potential. It thus causes a (sinus) bradycardia.
e. **True** – on stimulation the glomus cells of the chemoreceptor bodies release acetylcholine, among other neurotransmitters.

30 Answers

a. **True** – a catechol is a benzene ring with 2 hydroxyl groups (cx. 'phenol' which is a benzene ring with only one hydroxyl group). 'Catecholamine' is catechol attached to an (ethyl)amine moiety. The substitution in the case of adrenaline is: (i) a hydroxyl group on the β C atom; and (ii) a $- CH_3$ group on the $- NH_2 -$ the α C atom.
b. **False** – a quaternary ammonium compound is one that is a substituted $-NH_4^+$ group.
c. **False** – it is produced from noradrenaline by the insertion of a $-CH_3$ group (see **a.**)
d. **False** – 80%; the other 20% is noradrenaline.
e. **False** – noradrenaline is the major agonist.

31 Answers

a. **True**.
b. **True** – also in the medulla oblongata.
c. **True** – in fact they are found on most cholinergic nerve terminals and when activated inhibit the release of acetylcholine.
d. **True**.
e. **True** – their prototype antagonist is yohimbine. Prazosin is the prototype antagonist at α_1 receptor sites.

32 Answers

a. False – hypokalaemia is a manifestation of adrenergic agonism.

b. False – adrenergic stimulation causes a rise in blood sugar.

c. False – adrenergic agonism leads to lipolysis and a rise in blood free fatty acids.

d. True – because the levator palpebrae superioris muscle has a dual motor innervation: superior ramus of the oculomotor (3rd cranial) nerve and sympathetics from the superior cervical ganglion. Therefore the ptosis is partial and is a sign of Horner's syndrome (stellate ganglion block).

e. True – handling of viscera during abdominal surgery causes reflex firing of adrenergic inhibitory nerves, which inhibit the motor activity of the bowel and is regarded as the basis of postoperative ileus.

33 Answers

a. True – acebutolol is a selective β_1-adrenergic antagonist with some intrinsic sympathomimetic activity.

b. False – atenolol is a β_1-selective adrenergic antagonist that is devoid of intrinsic sympathomimetic activity.

c. False – esmolol is a β_1-selective adrenergic antagonist that has little, if any, intrinsic sympathomimetic activity, and it lacks membrane-stabilising actions.

d. True – pindolol is a non-subtype-selective β-adrenergic antagonist with intrinsic sympathomimetic activity.

e. False – propranolol is a non-selective pure β antagonist.

34 Answers

a. True.

b. False – the EW nucleus is a parasympathetic nucleus.

c. False – stellate ganglion block will lead to miosis.

d. False – pilocarpine is a pupillary constrictor.

e. True – ecothiopate is an irreversible inhibitor of acetylcholinesterase because it combines with the enzyme at its serine site.

35 Answers

a. False.

b. True.

c. True.

d. False.

e. True – unless H_2 receptor antagonists are administered concurrently.

Answers

a. **False** – EDRF may be nitric oxide or a related compound nitrosothiol. Also, the term 'nitric oxide' is used generically to refer to NO when produced by both constitutive and induced NO synthase, while EDRF is confined to NO when produced by constitutive NO synthase alone.

b. **False** – via guanosine monophosphate (GMP) from guanosine triphosphate.

c. **False** – its release is increased by calcium ions.

d. **True**.

e. **True**.

37 **Answers**

a. **False** – is also found in adults.

b. **True** – it is also found at the nape of the neck and along the great vessels of the thorax and abdomen.

c. **True**.

d. **False** – has a rich β-adrenergic innervation.

e. **True**.

Note: Brown fat is very rich in mitochondria, the inner membrane of which contains *thermogenin*, an uncoupling protein, which 'short-circuits' the mitochondria protein battery. By this mechanism heat rather than chemical energy is produced.

38 **Answers**

a. **True** – it has no units because it is a ratio: the volume of CO_2 produced to that of O_2 consumed.

b. **True** – it is a measurement over a period of time, as opposed to the respiratory exchange ratio (R), which is the ratio of the CO_2 produced to O_2 consumed at any given time.

c. **True** – because when carbohydrates are the sole metabolic substrate an equal volume of CO_2 is produced for each volume of O_2 consumed:

$$C_6H_{12}O_6 + 6O_2 = 6CO_2 + 6H_2O$$

Therefore the RQ is 1.0. With fat metabolism there is less CO_2 produced to that of O_2 consumed. Therefore the RQ is < 1.0.

d. **False** – the heart normally uses fat as well as carbohydrate as its energy substrates, while the brain's normal metabolic substrate is almost entirely glucose.

e. **False** – The RQ is a steady-state measurement and therefore cannot logically be considered to apply to a period of severe exercise. It is the *respiratory exchange ratio* that is strictly pertinent to severe exercise and that may reach a value of about 2.0 during severe exercise. This is because CO_2 is being blown off and lactic acid, from anaerobic glycolysis, is being converted to CO_2.

39   Answers

a. True – zinc is part of the active site of the enzyme and the zinc ion polarises the carbonyl group of ethyl alcohol which is then converted to acetaldehyde.

b. False.

c. True – the binding of water to zinc in carbonic anhydrase reduces the pKa of water from 15.7 to 7 and at this pKa the formation of hydroxide ions is facilitated, which then combine with CO_2 to form bicarbonate.

d. False.

e. True – the enzyme contains, among other moieties, a C I domain, which contains a pair of zinc ions and it is this domain that binds diacylglycerol.

40   Answers

a. True – it is absorbed down a concentration gradient.

b. True – although the agent is metabolised predominantly in the liver.

c. True.

d. True – it produces vasodilatation, which increases renal perfusion and increases diuresis.

e. False – also because first-pass metabolism of alcohol by the stomach is about 50% less in women because the alcohol dehydrogenase activity of the gastric mucosa is lower than in men.

41   Answers

a. True.

b. True.

c. True.

d. True.

e. False – it increases the amount of NO synthase and therefore of nitric oxide, which is one cause of vasodilatation after ethanol.

42   Answers

a. False – ANP is a 28-amino acid peptide.

b. False – despite its name, ANP is also secreted by the cardiac ventricles as well as the brain and vascular endothelium. In the case of the brain: natriuretic peptide B; vascular endothelium: natriuretic peptide C.

c. True.

d. False – it produces its effect by activation of guanylyl cyclase.

e. True.

43   **Answers**

 a. **True** – the O-H bond of a water molecule is strongly polarised because of the high electronegativity of oxygen, leading to a partial positive charge on the H atom and a partial negative charge on the oxygen atom. As a result the hydrogen atoms of one water molecule are strongly attracted to the oxygen atoms of other water molecules. This form of attraction is called *hydrogen bonding*.
 b. **True** – surface tension (milli-newtons per metre at room temperature: water: 73; chloroform: 27; ether: 17; olive oil: 32.)
 c. **True** – because it has a high boiling point (100°C) compared with most other fluids.
 d. **True** – 1 cal (4.2 J) per gram.
 e. **False** – high: c. 580 cal/g.

44   **Answers**

 a. **True** – the pHs of the four solutions are as follows: 5% Glucose: c. 4; Hartmann's solution: c.6–6.5; N-saline: c. 5; G-Saline: c. 4.5.

Note: the pHs vary slightly depending on the mode of manufacture of the different solutions.

 b. **False** – see **a**.
 c. **True** – all the water in a litre of 5% Glucose is free water. Free water is the water content of a solution that is not matched by an equivalent ionic concentration to make it iso-osmolar with plasma. The free water content of Glucose-saline is about 800 ml/L of solution. Hartmann's solution and N-Saline are regarded as having no free water. In strict logic, even Hartmann's solution and N-Saline have a small amount of free water because they too are slightly hypo-osmolar compared with plasma.
 d. **False** – Glucose–Saline has one-fifth the sodium content of N-Saline.
 e. **False** – they all have a real osmolarity in the range 278–285, but the calculated osmolarity of N-Saline is 308 mmol/L (i.e. 154 × 2), 154 being the number of millimoles each of sodium and chloride.

Note: 'calculated' osmolarity is a mathematical derivative. It is equivalent to the total number of discrete entities (ions, atoms or molecules) of solute that are possible in the solution. The 'real' osmolarity is what is actually measured and depends on the degree of ionisation of any ionisable entities. For instance, in the case of Normal Saline, since only about seven-eighths of the sodium chloride is dissociated, the real osmolarity is about 280 compared with the calculated osmolarity of 308 mosmol/L.

45 Answers

a. False – it contains 29 mmol of *sodium lactate* as buffer.
b. False – it contains 2 mmol (i.e. 4 milliequivalents) of calcium.
c. True – 5 mmol × 39 (atomic mass of potassium) = c. 200 mg.
d. True – depending on the commercial preparation.
e. False – it will distribute itself into the interstitial compartment (IT) because of a *hydrostatic pressure* gradient.

46 Answers

a. False – branched chain polysaccharides of sucrose by action of *Leuconostoc mesenteroides*.
b. False – they improve peripheral blood flow by reducing viscosity.
c. True.
d. True – the received view is that it does adversely affect Factor VIII activity.
e. True – because it interferes with the antigens on the surface of red cells, which are oligosaccharides.

47 Answers

a. False – it is degraded gelatin (polygeline), but of a molecular weight of c. 30 kDa.
b. False – it is a half-litre pack, but of 3.5% gelatin.
c. True – the chloride concentration is 145 mmol/L. Na^+: 145; K^+: 2.55; Ca^+: 3.15.
d. True – therefore it ought not to be infused directly via the same giving set before or after blood.
e. True – the pH is 7.3 + or − 0.3.

48 Answers

a. True.
b. True.
c. True – 7.4 + or − 0.3.
d. True – Na^+: 145 mmol L^{-1}; Cl^-: 120 mmol L^{-1}.
e. True.

49 Answers

a. False – they are branched compounds because they are obtained from amylopectin, a highly branched starch compound.
b. False – the greater the solubility.
c. True.
d. True – 30 ml of water per gram of the agent; gelatins: c. 15 ml of water per gram.
e. True.

a. **True** – the electrolytes are the main determinant of plasma osmolarity and sodium accounts for about 45% of the total ion concentration.
b. **True** – because of the Gibbs–Donnan effect arising from the presence of a much higher concentration of 'non-permeable' negatively charged osmoles, i.e. plasma proteins (c. 80 g/L) in the plasma compartment compared with that (c. 20–25 g/L) in the interstitial compartment.
c. **False** – the prime determinant of ECF volume is the total *amount* of extracellular sodium. The plasma sodium *concentration* is the main determinant of the *intracellular* volume.
d. **True** – because it is the key determinant of plasma osmolarity (see **a.**)
e. **False** – plasma sodium: 130–140 mmol/L. Sodium concentration of N-saline: 154 mmol/L.

51 Answers

a. **True** – its highest tonicity is only 70% of that of plasma.
b. **True** – bicarbonate concentration in mmol/L: saliva: 60–80; bile: 10–20; pancreatic juice: 70–100; small intestine: 25–30; large intestine: bicarbonate is actively secreted into the large intestine.
c. **True** – c. 8.0–8.3.
d. **False** – see **b** above.
e. **False** – chloride content of gastric juice: c. 155–175 mmol/L.

52 Answers

a. **True**.
b. **False** – the net sodium reabsorption is highest in the jejunum.
c. **False** – luminal contents have about the same concentration of Na^+ as the plasma. Na^+ absorption occurs without the need for a significant net concentration gradient because of the efficiency of the Na^+–K^+–ATPase pump at the baso-lateral membrane.
d. **True** – movement of Na^+ down its electrochemical potential provides the energy for movement of sugars and amino acids. Therefore the absorption of the latter two substances is an example of secondary active co-transport.
e. **True** – it is a primary active process dependent on the Na^+–K^+–ATPase pump.

53 **Answers**

a. **False** – practically all the water will be absorbed.

b. **False** – all water movement across body fluid compartment interfaces is passive and dependent on hydrostatic and/or osmolar gradients.

c. **False** – there is an immediate response by the pituitary, to the reduction in plasma osmolarity, by suppression of ADH release but the diuresis is delayed for about 20 minutes until any circulating ADH is inactivated.

d. **True** – because there is a Na^+–K^+–ATPase pump at the basal (as well as the lateral) membrane of the gut cell.

e. **False** – the movement of water as between the ICF and the ECF is essentially dependent on an osmolar gradient resulting from the activity of the Na^+–K^+–ATPase pump, which by keeping Na^+ out will also keep the water out.

54 **Answers**

a. **True** – this is the definition of 'anion gap'. It can also be defined as the difference between the 'ignored' or 'unmeasured' anions and cations in the plasma.

b. **True** – see **a** and **e**.

c. **False** – if there is bicarbonate loss then the kidney will retain chloride and therefore the measured anions in the plasma will be about the same. Similarly, in chloride excess there will be a mEq to mEq replacement of bicarbonate by chloride and therefore the anion gap remains essentially the same.

d. **True** – the negative charges on the plasma proteins account for the 'missing' anions in the anion gap. Therefore a fall in plasma albumin will lead to a lower anion gap.

e. **True** – in addition to being equal to the difference between measured cations and anions, the anion gap is also equal to the difference between *unmeasured* anions and cations:

anion gap = unmeasured anions – unmeasured cations

Thus an increase in anion gap can be produced by a fall in unmeasured cations (as in hypocalcaemia, hypokalaemia, hypomagnesaemia) or, more importantly, by a rise in unmeasured anions.

55 Answers

a. False – a normal pH may indicate a normal acid-base state or a fully compensated acid-base derangement.

b. False – only if the person is breathing atmospheric air, i.e. with an FiO_2 of c. 20%. But if the person is underventilating and the consequent hypoxia has been corrected by increasing the FiO_2, then the pO_2 may be normal or even higher, despite the continuing underventilation.

c. True – to have a normal paO_2 (when breathing air FiO_2 21%) and a normal $paCO_2$ there must be normoventilation.

d. False – it may indicate a respiratory acidosis. A raised *standard* bicarbonate indicates a metabolic alkalosis.

e. True.

56 Answers

a. False – there is a rise in the total bicarbonate, but not in the standard bicarbonate. The 'standard bicarbonate' is that bicarbonate level that would prevail if the pCO_2 were normal, i.e. under conditions of normocapnia.

b. False – the curve is shifted to the right.

c. False – the kidney cannot correct an *acute* respiratory acidosis by excreting acid.

d. False – the kidney cannot respond effectively to an *acute* respiratory acidosis.

e. False – the rationale of giving sodium bicarbonate in a metabolic acidosis is to convert it into a respiratory acidosis. Therefore it is illogical to give it in an attempt to correct a respiratory acidosis.

57 Answers

a. False – the pKa is 6.1, which in logarithmic terms is far removed from the pH of the plasma, which is 7.4.

b. True.

c. True – i.e. the lungs and the kidneys.

d. True – i.e. carbon dioxide.

e. True.

58 Answers

a. True – at a pCO_2 of 40 mmHg (5.3 kPa) and since the solubility coefficient of CO_2 is 0.03 mmol/L per mmHg at 37°C, the amount of dissolved CO_2 is 1.2 mmol/L.

b. False – as carbaminohaemoglobin, which accounts for about 1.0 ml of CO_2 per litre of arterial blood. Carboxyhaemoglobin results when carbon monoxide combines with haemoglobin.

c. True – but the amount of CO_2 carried as carbonic acid is extremely small, only c. 0.0017 mmol/L.

d. True – c. 70% of CO_2 carriage is in the form of HCO_3.

e. True – a small amount in combination with the amino acids of plasma proteins.

59 **Answers**

a. False – the process is one of 'oxygenation'. Oxidation involves the addition of protons or the removal of electrons. Oxygenation is the addition of oxygen. Oxidation in the case of haemoglobin would result in the formation of ferric iron and therefore of methaemoglobin.
b. False – a homotropic positive cooperative effect.
c. False.
d. False – an increase.
e. True – see **b**. above: a homotropic positive cooperative effect.

60 **Answers**

a. False – the red colour is due to the presence of methene bridges in the haem moiety.
b. True – essentially the histidine groups of the globin chains.
c. True – the CO_2 combines with the $-NH_2$ moieties of the amino acids to form carbamino groups.
d. True – in thalassaemia the alpha or beta chains of the globin moiety are replaced by gamma chains.
e. False – the fault is in the haem moiety.

61 **Answers**

a. False – although the presence of 2,3 diphosphoglycerate influences the binding of oxygen with haemoglobin, it does not act as an enzyme in the process.
b. False.
c. False.
d. False.
e. False – the reaction is non-enzyme-dependent and is irreversible and therefore the level of glycosylated haemoglobin is a more accurate indicator of the diabetic state than the blood sugar level.

62 **Answers**

a. False.
b. False – the P_{50} is lower because the HbO_2 dissociation curve is shifted to the left.
c. True – in sulphaemoglobinaemia the HbO_2 dissociation curve is shifted to the right.
d. False.
e. True – because of the shift of the HbO_2 dissociation curve to the right as a result of the chronic anaemia.

a. **True** – at a saturation of 96% the arterial pO_2 has to be c. 13–14 kPa.

b. **False** – it wouldn't be. If the patient were underventilating and the ensuing hypoxaemia had been corrected by means of supplementary oxygen, the arterial pCO_2 would be raised. If, however, the patient was breathing room air, then an SpO_2 of 96% must mean the ventilation is adequate and therefore the arterial pCO_2 would be within normal limits.

c. **False** – an SpO_2 of 96% simply means that whatever the haemoglobin concentration in the blood 96% of it is carrying oxygen. To ensure sufficient oxygen availability for bodily needs there must also be an adequate concentration of Hb.

d. **False** – if, for instance, the patient was suffering from cyanide poisoning, the SpO_2 could be normal, but because of the effect of cyanide on cytochrome oxidase the tissues would be unable to utilise oxygen and thus would suffer hypoxia.

e. **False** – in carbon monoxide poisoning the ensuing carboxyhaemoglobinaemia leads to an SpO_2 reading of c. 96%, no matter the actual haemoglobin oxygen saturation.

64 Answers

a. **True**.

b. **False** – is produced in the Rapaport–Leubering shunt of the Embden–Meyerhof glycolytic pathway.

c. **True**.

d. **False** – is bound to the β chain of the haemoglobin molecule.

e. **False** – is present in a concentration of 1 molecule per molecule of haemoglobin.

65   Answers

a. **True** – the relationship between haematocrit and viscosity is direct and in the form of an accelerating exponential. At lower haematocrits viscosity is dependent on red cell 'stickiness'; at higher viscosities it is dependent on red cell deformation.

b. **True** – the main reason for the variation of viscosity with the level of fibrinogen (i.e. the non-newtonian behaviour of blood) is the interaction of fibrinogen with red cells. Thus plasma (which contains fibrinogen but no red cells) is newtonian, and so is a suspension of washed red cells in saline (i.e. devoid of fibrinogen).

c. **True** – viscosity of a fluid is inversely related to temperature.

d. **True** – in larger vessels radius > 1 mm in diameter blood viscosity is independent of vessel calibre. However, at lower radii the blood viscosity decreases steeply due to a phenomenon called the Fahraeus–Lindqvist effect. It begins to appear when vessel diameter falls below c. 1.5 mm and is due to the red cells, which instead of moving randomly, align themselves in a single line as they pass along the vessel.

e. **True** – the higher the linear velocity, the lower the viscosity, because blood is a *thixotropic* fluid. Its viscosity is related to its shear rate, which in turn is dependent on its flow rate.

66   Answers

a. **True**.

b. **False** – the A and B red cell antigens are oligosaccharides; it is tissue antigens that are glycoproteins.

c. **False** – predominantly IgG and IgM antibodies.

d. **True** – also called an O antigen.

e. **False** – the antigens of the donor blood combine with the antibodies of the recipient red cells.

Note: the common structural foundation of the antigens is an oligosaccharide called the O or H antigen, which is the one present in group O individuals. The A and B antigens have an additional monosaccharide, either N-acetylgalactosamine (for A) or galactose (for B).

67   Answers

a. **True** – but note that von Willebrand's disease takes several different forms with different inheritance patterns, but the main form of inheritance is autosomal dominant.

b. **False** – it is sex-linked recessive.

c. **False** – it is sex-linked recessive.

d. **False** – it is autosomal recessive.

e. **False** – it is autosomal recessive.

a. **False** – it occurs when carbon dioxide combines with haemoglobin.
b. **False** – the combination is with the histidine residues of the globin moiety of the haemoglobin molecule.
c. **False** – unlike the combination of CO_2 with water to form H_2CO_3, which is dependent on carbonic anhydrase, carbaminohaemoglobin formation requires no enzyme.
d. **False** – only 20–25% of CO_2 is carried in the blood as carbaminohaemoglobin. Most (c. 65%) is carried as bicarbonate.
e. **True** – the Hamburger phenomenon is the 'chloride shift' that follows formation of bicarbonate, a phenomenon that occurs concurrently with the formation of carbaminohaemoglobin.

69 Answers

a. **True** – infection with *Pneumocystis carinii* can occur in AIDS patients, and primaquine, given for treatment of AIDS, is the cause of the methaemoglobinaemia.
b. **True** – it results from the administration of prilocaine for Bier's block.
c. **True**.
d. **True** – the condition biases the SpO_2 reading towards c. 85%, no matter the true oxygen saturation level.
e. **True** – methylene blue can cause haemolysis in a dosage of > 15 g/kg.

70 Answers

a. **True**.
b. **True**.
c. **False**.
d. **True**.
e. **False** – if at all, the curve may be displaced to the right because of the anaemia commonly associated with the condition.

71 Answers

a. **True** – because of production of metabolic acids (pyruvic and lactic acids) from glycolysis, which although diminished because of the lowered temperature nevertheless continues.
b. **True** – because at $4°C$ the $Na^+–K^+–ATPase$ pump is markedly inhibited and therefore both sodium and potassium moves down their respective concentration gradients, leading to a rise in plasma potassium and a fall in plasma sodium.
c. **True** – see **b**.
d. **False** – because of reduced glycolysis. 2,3 diphosphoglycerate is formed in the Rapaport–Luebering shunt of the glycolytic (Embden–Meyerhof) pathway. Reduction in the temperature of stored blood reduces glycolysis and thus leads to a lower level of 2,3 DPG.
e. **True**.

72   Answers

a. **True**.
b. **True**.
c. **False** – it increases clotting factors by c. 2–3% per 'unit' transfused.
d. **True**.
e. **False** – it is desirable but not mandatory to ensure ABO compatibility.

73   Answers

a. **True** – because they do not have nuclei.
b. **False** – lifespan of platelets: 10–12 days; of leucocytes: a few hours in the peripheral circulation and c. 4–5 days in the tissues.
c. **True**.
d. **True**.
e. **False** – as their name suggests, leukotrienes are eicosanoids with three unsaturated carbon bonds (hence, *triene*) found in white cells (hence *leuko*). They are not present in platelets, which have thromboxane A_2.

74   Answers

a. **True**.
b. **False**.
c. **False** – it is not necessary to be ABO compatible.
d. **False** – they must be transfused within 4 hours of being pooled.
e. **False** – must not be given until the splenic pedicle has been tied off.

75   Answers

a. **True** – the process is explosive in nature.
b. **False** – the rate-limiting factor is the formation of prothrombin activator (PTa).
c. **True** – prothrombin attaches itself to prothrombin receptors on platelets that are already bound to damaged endothelium in the process of conversion into thrombin.
d. **False** – Ca^{2+} has several roles in the coagulation process: (i) accelerates activation of Factor X by Factor IXa; (ii) converts prothrombin to thrombin; and (iii) converts fibrin monomers to fibrin fibres.
e. **True**.

a. **True** – vitamins A, D, E and K are fat soluble.
b. **True** – but it is not the body's main source of vitamin K. There are two forms of vitamin K: phylloquinone, which is found in plants and is obtained from plant food, and menaquinone, which is produced by *Escherichia coli* in the intestine. The latter is not the primary source of the body's vitamin K.
c. **False** – its activity occurs in the rough endoplasmic reticulum of hepatocytes.
d. **False** – it is required to carboxylate glutamate residues in the coagulation factors II, VII, IX and X to γ – carboxyglutamate. It is the γ - carboxyglutamate that confers Ca^{2+} binding properties on the coagulation factors, in other words coverts them from their 'precursor' form to their active form.
e. **False** – by being prevented from undergoing reduction. Carboxylation of glutamate by vitamin K is associated with oxidation of the vitamin to vitamin K epoxide. It is the enzymatic re-conversion of vitamin K epoxide to vitamin K, a reduction reaction, that is blocked by warfarin.

77   **Answers**

a. **False** – because the warfarin is less protein bound, it is more free to be broken down and therefore has a shorter half-life.
b. **False** – the action is shortened because of enzyme induction.
c. **False** – because of increased levels of coagulation factors.
d. **True** – because of destruction of gut bacteria, resulting in less vitamin K formation.
e. **True** – cephalosporins inhibit vitamin K epoxidase.

78   **Answers**

a. **True** – the fundamental aim of the cardiac ventricle as a pump is to generate a constant blood pressure, and under normal physiological conditions the body does this essentially by altering the peripheral vascular resistance.
b. **False** – almost 95% of the energy expenditure is to pump blood against a pressure gradient, and only a small amount of energy is expended to impart kinetic motion to the blood.
c. **False** – the right ventricles contract like a bellows, its free wall moving towards the interventricular septum, while in the case of the left ventricle the constriction of its circular muscle from apex to base is akin to a hand squeezing a tube of toothpaste.
d. **False** – contraction starts slightly earlier in the case of the left ventricle.
e. **False** – right ventricular ejection lasts slightly longer than that of the left ventricle.

79   Answers

a. **True** – due to a rapid increase in Na⁺ conductance.
b. **True** – and also closure of sodium channels.
c. **True** – prolonged opening of voltage-gated Ca^{2+} channels.
d. **True** – it is due to closure of voltage-gated Ca^{2+} channels and K⁺ efflux through two kinds of K⁺ channels.
e. **False** – mainly dependent on K⁺ conductivity of cell membrane.

80   Answers

a. **True**.
b. **True**.
c. **True**.
d. **True**.
e. **True**.

81   Answers

a. **False** – there is little, if any, parasympathetic innervation of the ventricles.
b. **False** – the M_2 type.
c. **False** – T1–4.
d. **True**.
e. **True**.

82   Answers

a. **True**.
b. **True**.
c. **True**.
d. **True**.
e. **False**.

83   Answers

a. **True** – this is in conformity with Starling's law of the heart.
b. **True** – so as to bring the ventricular end-diastolic blood volume back to normal.
c. **True** – results from the increase in blood pressure that would result from **a** and **b**.
d. **False** – the carotid body is concerned with chemoreceptor activity, not baroreceptor activity, except at very high blood pressures.
e. **False** – the Bainbridge reflex – tachycardia as a result of increased venous return – is mediated via stretch receptors in the atrium and not ventricular muscle fibre stretching.

84   Answers

a. **True** – because part of the recipient's right atrium is normally left behind.
b. **False** – it has a low-normal cardiac output.
c. **False** – it has an increased response from increased sensitivity resulting from denervation.
d. **False** – occurs usually in the first 3 months.
e. **True** – because of non-sensitivity of myocardium arising from denervation.

85   Answers

a. **False** – it is due to atrial contraction regurgitating some blood upwards into the jugular vein (as well as propelling blood into the right ventricle).
b. **False** – it is the a-wave that is almost synchronous with the 1st heart sound.
c. **False** – a 'cannon wave' is an exaggerated a-wave.
d. **True** – although the vein itself may be prominent, its waves are not so prominent because the vein is nipped by the thickened pericardium during ventricular systole.
e. **True**.

86   Answers

a. **False** – the pulse pressure wave is faster: $3–14$ m s^{-1}, c. $15–100$ times the blood flow rate.
b. **True**.
c. **False** – velocity of pressure pulse transmission: in aorta: $3–5$ m s^{-1}; in large arteries: $7–10$ ms^{-1}; in small arteries: $15–35$ m s^{-1}.
d. **False**.
e. **False**.

87   Answers

a. **False** – a falsely low reading is likely because the arm pressure would be lower by a factor equal to the height of the arm above heart level.
b. **True**.
c. **True** – but not just because the mercury reservoir is below cuff level, but because the zero reference point of the Hg column, to which the Hg reservoir level is referenced, is below cuff level.
d. **False** – a wider cuff is more likely to give a falsely low reading.
e. **False** – more likely to give a falsely lower reading.

88 Answers

a. **True**.
b. **True**.
c. **True**.
d. **True**.
e. **True**.

Note: Turbulence is dependent on the critical value for Reynolds' number:

$$Re = d \, v \times \rho/\eta$$

Where d = diameter of vessel wall; v = velocity of flow; ρ = density of fluid; η = viscosity of fluid.

89 Answers

a. **True** – c. 100 mmHg compared with c. 50 mmHg for the aortic baroreceptors.
b. **False** – higher.
c. **True**.
d. **False** – they are less sensitive.
e. **True**.

90 Answers

a. **False** – O_2 consumption in ml per 100 g tissue: brain: 3.5; heart: 8.5; liver: 3.5; kidneys: 7.0; adrenals: c. 30–40 ml.
b. **True** – two-thirds in diastole, one-third in systole. None of the other organs has such a wide discrepancy between blood flow in the two phases of systole and diastole.
c. **True** – adrenal glands: mass c. 8–10 g; blood flow: c. 20–25 ml. Therefore blood flow is c. 300–500 ml per 100 g tissue. Note: the organ with the highest blood flow is the carotid body: c. 2000 ml per 100 g.
d. **False** – Liver: 1400 ml, i.e. 28%; kidneys: 1200 ml, i.e. 24%.
e. **True** – because most of the blood to the liver is via the portal vein, which already has a lower O_2 content than arterial blood. Portal vein oxygen: c.12 ml per 100 ml blood.

91 Answers

a. **False** – is striated just like skeletal muscle.
b. **True**.
c. **True** – fast sodium channels (just like skeletal muscle) and slow calcium channels, also known as Ca-Na channels (which skeletal muscle does not have).
d. **True** – cardiac muscle: about 4–6 kg cm^{-2}. Skeletal muscle: about 3–4 kg cm^{-2}.
e. **True** – one-tenth that of skeletal muscle.

Answers

a. **True**.
b. **False** – the commonest aetiological factor is atherosclerosis.
c. **False** – shows no symptoms until the disease is advanced.
d. **True** – for reasons stated in **b**.
e. **True** – in fact it is the only valvular lesion that is associated with anaesthetic morbidity and mortality.

Answers

a. **True** – probe-patent foramen ovale is found in c. 25% of postmortem subjects.
b. **False** – it is rarely symptomatic during childhood.
c. **True**.
d. **True** – for the same reason as in **a**.
e. **True**.

Answers

a. **True**.
b. **True**.
c. **False** – can occur even if the endothelium is damaged.
d. **True** – thus enabling blood to be shunted away from the non-aerating lung.
e. **True**.

Answers

a. **True** – the cerebral blood flow is 750 ml/minute and the $CMRO_2$ is 50 ml/minute. Therefore every 100 ml of blood [Hb 15 g] has about 750/50, i.e. 7 ml of O_2 removed from it, leaving 13 ml. Therefore the Hb saturation is 13/20, i.e. about 65%. The mixed venous O_2 saturation is 75%.
b. **True** – coronary blood flow: c. 220 ml/minute; cardiac oxygen consumption: c. 26 ml/minute. Therefore the oxygen extraction is c. 26/2.2, i.e. 12 ml per 100 ml of blood. Therefore the coronary venous blood has an oxygen content of 20 minus 12 ml, i.e. 8 ml O_2 per 100 ml of blood. Therefore the O_2 saturation is c. 40%.
c. **True** – portal vein blood normally has an oxygen content of c. 12 ml per 100 ml; Hb 15 g/100 ml. Therefore the hepatic vein blood must have less than that, i.e. less than that of mixed venous blood.
d. **False** – renal oxygen consumption: c. 20 ml min^{-1}; renal blood flow: c. 1200 ml min^{-1}. Therefore the oxygen extraction is 20/12, i.e. c. 1. 7 ml per 100 ml of blood. Therefore renal vein blood has 18.3 ml O_2 per 100 ml, i.e. c. 92%.
e. **False** – it is about the same as mixed venous blood.

96 Answers

a. True – because the physiological dead space is the sum of the anatomical and alveolar dead spaces, and there is virtually no alveolar dead space in the healthy young adult person.

b. True – because the alveolar capillary membrane is extremely efficient.

c. True – the 'standard bicarbonate' is that bicarbonate level a person would have under the 'standard' condition of a normal pCO_2.

d. False – liver blood flow: c. 100 ml per 100 g tissue; cerebral blood flow: c. 55 ml per 100 g.

e. False – total resting cardiac oxygen consumption: c. 26 ml/minute; total cerebral oxygen consumption: c. 50 ml/minute.

97 Answers

a. False – hepatic blood flow: c. 1500 ml/minute; weight of the liver: c. 1500 g. Therefore blood flow: c. 100 ml per 100 g/minute. Heart: blood flow: c. 220 ml/minute; weight: c. 300 g. Therefore blood flow: c. 75 ml per 100 g/minute.

b. True – brain weight: c. 1400 g; oxygen consumption: c. 50 ml/minute. Therefore oxygen consumption per 100 g: c. 3.5 ml/minute. Heart: weight c. 300 g; oxygen consumption: c. 26 ml/minute. Therefore oxygen consumption per 100 g: c. 8.5 ml/minute.

c. False – the heart uses mainly fats as its energy substrate, glucose only accounting for less than half. Red blood cells use glucose exclusively as their substrate because they do not have mitochondria.

d. True – c. 1 W compared with c. 0.625 W for breathing.

The work of breathing: (approximate) = tidal volume × mean pressure change = $0.5 \times 10^{-3} \times 2.5 \times 10^3$ joules 0.5 W = 0.625 W

Work of cardiac contraction: (approximate) = $75 \times 10^{-6} \times 13.3 \times 10^3$ W = 1 W.

e. False – heart: c. 3%; respiration: c. 5%.

98 Answers

a. False – the terminal bronchioles allow gas exchange through their walls and, therefore, by definition are not part of the anatomical dead space, which therefore ends just 'proximal' to the terminal bronchioles.

b. True – see also **c**.

c. False – the neonate has a V_T of c. 16 ml and a V_D of c. 5 ml, therefore the ratio is c. 0.3, which is about the same as in an adult.

d. True – orotracheal intubation removes about 70 ml from the anatomical dead space.

e. False – its measurement is done by use of a rapid gas analyser, which plots the 'alveolar plateau' of CO_2 concentration and the dead space is derived from the resulting graph.

Answers

a. **True**.
b. **False** – see **e** of previous MCQ.
c. **False** – residual volume can be determined by measuring either Functional residual capacity (FRC) or expiratory reserve volume by a nitrogen washout technique and then deriving the residual volume from the obtained figure.
d. **False** – determination of the physiological dead space requires measurement of the pCO_2 of mixed expired air and arterial blood and application of the Bohr equation.
e. **True**.

100 **Answers**

a. **True** – c. 150 ml.
b. **True**.
c. **True** – the final stage of gas movement, from terminal bronchioles to alveoli, is by simple diffusion.
d. **False** – the greatest resistance is in some of the larger bronchioles because there are fewer of them compared with about 65,000 terminal bronchioles.
e. **False** – no more than about 5%.

101 **Answers**

a. **False** – flow is intermittent. There is no flow in diastole.
b. **False**.
c. **False** – systolic pressure > alveolar pressure > diastolic pressure.
d. **False**.
e. **True**.

102 **Answers**

a. **True** – net pulmonary capillary transudation pressure is c. 7 mmHg compared with its systemic counterpart, which is c. 17 mmHg.
b. **True**.
c. **True**.
d. **False** – there are small openings between alveolar epithelial cells that can permit even large protein molecules to pass through.
e. **False**.

103 Answers

a. **False** – about half. 1/C of the combined L–T system = 1/C of the lungs + 1/C of the thorax. (Think of electrical resistances in parallel)
b. **True.**
c. **False** – it decreases to about one-fifth.
d. **True** – normal expiration is a passive process resulting from elastic recoil of the lungs, the energy for the process being that stored as potential energy in the chest wall during inspiration.
e. **False** – two-thirds.

104 Answers

a. **True.**
b. **False** – it reaches body temperature by the time it reaches the vocal cords.
c. **False** – by turbulent precipitation.
d. **False** – the particle size reaching the alveoli is less than 6 microns; red cell size c. 7–8 microns.
e. **False** – the cigarette smoke particle size is c. 1–3 microns, therefore they reach the alveoli.

105 Answers

a. **True.**
b. **True.**
c. **False** – it tends to fall because of hyperventilation secondary to hypoxia.
d. **False** – it increases as much as 3-fold from its normal value of 21 ml per mmHg pressure per minute.
e. **True** – as a compensatory measure.

106 Answers

a. **True** – it is c. 10–20% of total blood volume.
b. **False** – about 1–2% is received via the bronchial arterioles.
c. **False** – the pulmonary capillaries contain only about 100 ml of blood at any time; the rest is divided about equally between the arteries and the veins.
d. **True.**
e. **True.**

a. True – as well as Phase I biotransformations.
b. False – angiotensinogen is converted to angiotensin I in the plasma by renin. The conversion of angiotensin I to angiotensin II by ACE occurs in the lung (and elsewhere).
c. True – 98% of serotonin inactivation occurs in the lung.
d. False – mast cells are not manufactured by the pulmonary endothelium but by the subendothelial connective tissue cells of airways as well as alveolar septa.
e. False – arachidonic acid is not stored in the pulmonary endothelium; it is synthesised as required and immediately released into the circulation.

108 Answers

a. True.
b. False – Type II cells, which contain striated osmiophilic organelles that store the surfactant.
c. False – surfactant is a complex mixture and includes dipalmitoyl phosphatidyl choline (i.e. dipalmitoyl lecithin), other phospholipids, apoproteins and calcium ions.
d. False – forms in the 6th to 7th months of fetal life.
e. True – surface tension of water: c. 73 millinewtons per metre at room temperature.

109 Answers

a. True – by about 800 ml.
b. True.
c. True.
d. False – oesophageal sphincter tone is increased.
e. True.

110 Answers

a. False – mere hyperventilation will not significantly increase the alveolar pO_2 and therefore the arterial pO_2 above its normal of c. 13–14 kPa unless there is also an increase in the FiO_2.
b. True – the resulting respiratory alkalosis will lead to hypokalemia, albeit a mild one.
c. False – the haemoglobin oxygen dissociation curve would be shifted to the left as a result of the respiratory alkalosis and therefore there will be a fall in the P_{50} of haemoglobin.
d. False – standard bicarbonate is the bicarbonate level a person would have if their pCO_2 were normal.
e. False – an acute respiratory alkalosis (or acidosis) does not produce a compensatory metabolic acidosis (or alkalosis) by excretion of alkaline (or acid) urine because the kidney cannot respond fast enough to such a change.

111 Answers

a. **False** – but noradrenaline is removed by the pulmonary endothelial cells.
b. **True**.
c. **False**.
d. **True**.
e. **False**.

112 Answers

a. **False** – c. 20–25%.
b. **True** – kidneys: 1200ml/minute; liver: 1400 ml/minute.
c. **False** – heart: c. 25 ml/minute; liver c. 50 ml/minute.
d. **True** – brain: 55 ml per 100 g of tissue; liver: 100 ml per 100 g of tissue.
e. **True** – adult: 2%; neonate: 5%.

113 Answers

a. **True** – c.10%; kidneys c. 90%.
b. **True**.
c. **False** – nitrous oxide is not known to be broken down in the body. It is excreted in its entirety via the lungs and to a very small extent through the skin.
d. **True** – it secretes it into the bile and from there into the gut; then it is excreted in the faeces.
e. **False** – urobilinogen is formed in the gut from bilirubin secreted into it from the liver.

114 Answers

a. **True**.
b. **False** – mast cells elsewhere, lung and intestine, also produce heparin.
c. **False** – the liver does not manufacture vitamin K. It is normally obtained in the diet as phylloquinone, and as menaquinone is produced by *Escherichia coli* in the intestine.
d. **True** – but the liver cannot break down ketones.
e. **False** – brain cells and red cells also can receive glucose without the need for insulin.

Answers

a. **False** – about 50% of the brain's cell volume.
b. **False** – about × 4: grey matter c. 75–80 ml per 100 g/minute; white matter c. 20 ml per 100 g/minute.
c. **True** – Total body basal oxygen consumption: 250 ml/minute; cerebral oxygen consumption: 50 ml/minute.
d. **True** – to maintain the transneuronal electrical gradient.
e. **False** – under normal conditions glucose accounts for 95% of the substrate; the rest is glutamate. Under hypoxic conditions the brain can use ketones as its metabolic substrate.

116 **Answers**

a. **False** – there is no evidence that clinically used anaesthetic concentrations adversely affect the BBB.
b. **True** – this has been observed, presumably the result of the rise in intracapillary hydrostatic pressure.
c. **True**.
d. **True**.
e. **False** – there is no evidence to this effect.

117 **Answers**

a. **False** – only occurs in necrosis. Cerebral cell shrinkage is the feature of apoptosis.
b. **True**.
c. **False** – only present in necrosis.
d. **True**.
e. **False** – only present in necrosis.

Note: Apoptosis is 'programmed cell death' and one of its hallmarks is the cleavage of chromosomal DNA into nucleosomal subunits. The degradation of DNA in apoptotic cell nuclei is accomplished following activation by *caspases*, a family of cysteine proteases that exist within cells as inactive pro-forms (zymogens). Nitric oxide is involved in regulating apoptosis. Depending on the type of cell and the dose of NO, the agent can induce apoptosis or protect cells from apoptosis.

118 **Answers**

a. **True** – it reduces CMR by 6–7% per °C of temperature reduction.
b. **False** – glucose in the absence of O_2 acts a substrate for anaerobic glycolysis, leading to a lactic acidosis, which aggravates the ischaemic injury.
c. **False** – hypercapnia: (i) aggravates acidosis; and (ii) has the potential to cause an intracerebral 'steal' phenomenon.
d. **True** – maintaining a raised blood pressure after ischaemic injury helps to maintain more even cerebral perfusion than normotension.
e. **False** – see **c** above.

119   Answers

   a. True – dependent on active transport of Na^+, which draws water into the subarachnoid space.

   b. True – the difference is about 4%.

   c. True.

   d. False – the volume of CSF is about 150 ml. The daily volume of CSF secreted is about 500 ml. Therefore the change is about 3–4 times per day.

   e. True.

120   Answers

   a. False – more than 50% is due to increases in mother's anatomy. The total increase is c. 10 kg. Fetus: c. 3 kg; amniotic fluid: c. 2.5 kg; maternal blood and uterus: c. 3 kg; uterus: 1 kg; breasts c.1 kg.

   b. False – the CO rises by c. 30–40% up to 27 weeks, then falls to just above normal in the last 8–10 weeks.

   c. True.

   d. False – it increases by about 15%, mainly in the second half of pregnancy.

   e. True – up by about 30%.

121   Answers

   a. False – gastric motility is reduced because of the effects of higher progesterone levels.

   b. True – because of increased vascularity of muscle tissue.

   c. False – renal blood flow is increased by about 50%, but hepatic flow remains essentially the same.

   d. True – because plasma albumin is reduced (from about 45 g/L to about 35g/L), although globulin increases by about 10% by term.

   e. False – cholinesterase activity is decreased, but it is of little clinical significance.

122   Answers

   a. True.

   b. True.

   c. True.

   d. True – consequent on c.

   e. True – it falls to c. 30–40 mg/dl.

123 **Answers**

   a. **False** – blood volume in the neonate is about 80–100 ml/kg; adult: about 70 ml/kg.
   b. **True** – adult: about 100 ml/kg; neonate: c. 200 ml/kg.
   c. **False** – the FRC is about half (in relation to body weight) of that of an adult.
   d. **True** – c. 150 ml/kg in the neonate; adult: c. 75 ml/kg.
   e. **True** – adult: 3.5 ml/kg; neonate: c. 7.0 ml/kg.

124 **Answers**

   a. **True**.
   b. **False** – the blood–brain barrier is more permeable.
   c. **True** – the adult, though absorbing water and electrolytes in the large bowel, has virtually no absorption of dietary nutrients through it.
   d. **False** – drug absorption is slower because gastric emptying is slower and intestinal transit time is longer.
   e. **False** – rectal absorption of drugs is much more efficient in the neonate than in the adult.

125 **Answers**

   a. **True**.
   b. **True**.
   c. **False** – it is gender-linked recessive.
   d. **False** – it is X-linked recessive. However, this is a misnomer because it is possible to be 'heterozygous' for the abnormality, and a recessive trait is, by definition, not expressed in a heterozygote.
   e. **False** – it is autosomal recessive.

126 **Answers**

   a. **True**.
   b. **True** – children: 1 in 12,000; adults: 1 in 40,000.
   c. **True**.
   d. **False** – a rise in end-tidal CO_2 is usually the first sign.
   e. **False** – there is a combined respiratory acidosis (from a rise in CO_2 production) and a metabolic acidosis (from tissue hypoxia).

127 **Answers**

   a. **False** – it can sometimes be acquired.
   b. **True**.
   c. **False** – it is worsened by smoking.
   d. **True**.
   e. **True** – severe hyponatraemia may be present because of the syndrome of inappropriate ADH secretion.

128 Answers

a. **False** – it is an autosomal dominant condition.
b. **False** – normally presents in the third to fourth decades.
c. **False** – the increase is in *creatine* kinase levels.
d. **False** – it is improved by Class I antiarrhythmics such as phenytoin and procainamide.
e. **False** – it is made worse by pregnancy.

129 Answers

a. **True**.
b. **True**.
c. **True**.
d. **True**.
e. **True**.

130 Answers

a. **True** – from hypoprothrombinaemia due to a warfarin-like action on the vitamin K epoxide cycle.
b. **True**.
c. **True** – by increasing O_2 consumption by uncoupling oxidative phosphorylation.
d. **True** – rare but possible.
e. **False** – may occur but later.

131 Answers

a. **True** – because of the fixed cardiac output the person tries to maintain blood pressure by increasing the systemic vascular resistance.
b. **False** – it rises (Kussmaul's sign) because of the constricting effect on the 'base' of the vein by the pericardium.
c. **True**.
d. **False** – the V-wave is lacking because there is no significant tricuspid regurgitation.
e. **True** – an early diastolic sound, whose timing is related to the end of rapid ventricular filling but heard slightly earlier than the classic 3rd heart sound.

132 Answers

a. **True**.
b. **False**.
c. **False** – hypothyroidism is the more likely condition.
d. **False** – relatively common.
e. **True**.

133 Answers

a. **False** – it is a postsynaptic membrane disorder.
b. **True**.
c. **True**.
d. **True** – see **a** above.
e. **True**.

134 Answers

a. **True**.
b. **False** – the abnormality is at the pre-synaptic membrane leading to a reduction in release of acetylcholine quanta, although each quantum is normal (cx. myasthenia gravis, where the abnormality is postsynaptic).
c. **False** – ocular involvement is rare (cx. myasthenia gravis).
d. **False** – it may precede appearance of the tumour by up to 2 years.
e. **False** – autonomic dysfunction is common.

135 Answers

a. **True**.
b. **True** – although it is more commonly acquired.
c. **True**.
d. **True** – there is increased velocity and therefore an increase in kinetic energy at the site of airway narrowing. Thus in accordance with the law of conservation of mechanical energy there is a decrease in potential (pressure) energy and therefore collapse of the pharyngeal muscles.
e. **False** – usually unaware.

136 Answers

a. **True**.
b. **True** – due to a unique form of myosin in the masseter muscle.
c. **True** – in about 50% of patients who develop malignant hyperpyrexia.
d. **True**.
e. **True**.

137 Answers

a. **True** – and the vagus is the efferent nerve.
b. **False** – it is more likely in children, especially during operations for strabismus.
c. **True** – bradycardia is more common but ventricular fibrillation is a distinct possibility.
d. **True** – retrobulbar blockade is a method of minimising the risks of the reflex being activated but can itself be the cause of it too.
e. **True**.

138 Answers

a. **False** – it decreases because body fat tends to increase and fat has a lower water content than lean tissue.
b. **False** – lung compliance is increased because of loss of lung elasticity.
c. **False** – although creatinine clearance may be reduced because of gradual impairment of renal function, the decrease in muscle mass means less creatinine is produced. Therefore the serum creatinine is essentially unchanged.
d. **True** – reduced by c. 4% per decade of age after 40 years.
e. **True.**

139 Answers

a. **False** – they can also be catalysed by plasma and tissue esterases.
b. **False** – almost exclusively.
c. **False** – conjugation reactions are Phase II biotransformations. Phase I biotransformations 'functionalise' drugs by producing or uncovering a chemically reactive functional group in the drugs on which Phase II reactions can take place.
d. **False** – leukotriene synthesis involves both Phase I and Phase II reactions.
e. **False** – the primary purpose is to moderately increase drug polarity and prepare it for Phase II activity, which latter markedly increases drug polarity and thus makes the drugs more easily excretable.

140 Answers

a. **False** – it is a Phase II process.
b. **False** – most conjugation processes occur in the cytosol, the exception being glucuronidation, which occurs in the endoplasmic reticulum.
c. **False**.
d. **False** – it renders drugs hydrophilic and thereby more easily excretable via the kidneys.
e. **True** – example: morphine, which is converted to morphine-6-glucuronide, a more potent analgesic than the parent compound.

a. **False** – Phase II.
b. **False** – it is a 'conjugation' reaction. The substrate is conjugated with a moiety, glucuronide, to make the agent highly polar and therefore easily excretable.
c. **False** – unlike most Phase II reactions, which are sited in the cytosol, glucuronidation takes place in the endoplasmic reticulum.
d. **False** – the enzyme responsible is uridine diphosphate (UDP)-glucuronosyltransferase.
e. **True** – morphine produces two metabolites from Phase II biotransformation: morphine 1 glucuronide and morphine 6 glucuronide: the latter is the active metabolite and is a more potent analgesic than the parent compound.

142 **Answers**

a. **True** – glucuronidation is a Phase II biotransformation reaction, one purpose of which is to make the agent more hydrophilic for easier renal excretion.
b. **False** – hydrocarbons are generally hydrophobic.
c. **False** – steroids are normally less hydrophilic.
d. **True**.
e. **True** – like glucuronidation, acetylation is a Phase II reaction, the purpose of which is to render the drug water soluble.

143 **Answers**

a. **True**.
b. **True**.
c. **True**.
d. **False** – no relationship to pharmacological activity.
e. **True**.

144 **Answers**

a. **True**.
b. **False** – it complexes with carbon *mono*xide. Note: the CO is not involved in the reaction; it merely gives a complex with a spectrum that makes it easy to measure the amount of P 450.
c. **False** – it is found in the smooth endoplasmic reticulum.
d. **False** – it is a mono-oxygenase system because it uses just one atom of oxygen from each oxygen molecule, the other being reduced to water by NADPH thus:

$$AH + O_2 + NADPH + H^+ = A\text{-}OH + H_2O + NADP.$$

e. **True** – because it has a 'mixed' or dual function; it both *hydroxylates* AH and *reduces* the other oxygen atom to H_2O. See equation under **d**.

145   Answers

a. False – propofol is a substituted phenol (2,6 di-isopropyl phenol).
b. True.
c. False – ketamine is a phencyclidine derivative.
d. True.
e. False – vasopressin is a nonapeptide.

146   Answers

a. True – morphine is an 'opiate' because it is obtained from opium, and an 'opioid' because it acts on opioid receptors.
b. True.
c. True.
d. True – atropine is tropic acid combined with tropine.
e. True – diclofenac is 'dichloro-anilino-phenyl-acetic acid.

147   Answers

a. False – adenosine is eliminated with a half-life of seconds by carrier-mediated uptake, which occurs in most cell types including capillary endothelium, and subsequent degradation by adenosine deaminase.
b. False – seconds. Adrenaline is rapidly inactivated in the body by: (i) re-uptake; and (ii) enzymatic degradation by monoamine oxidase (MAO) and catechol O-methyl transferase (COMT).
c. True – c. 20–30 minutes.
d. True – c. 5–6 minutes. It is destroyed primarily in the liver by insulinase.
e. False – seconds. It is rapidly inactivated by haemoglobin.

148   Answers

a. True – the process is dependent on vitamin D. Calcium is also absorbed throughout the small intestine by facilitated diffusion.
b. True – of the rest 10% is bound to citrate, phosphate, etc. and the rest to plasma proteins.
c. False – a direct relationship.
d. True.
e. True.

149   Answers

a. True.
b. True.
c. True.
d. True.
e. True – because angiotensin II is a kinase.

150 Answers

a. **False** – Xenon: MAC 71%; N_2O: MAC c. 105%.
b. **False** – Xenon has a density of c. 5.88 g/L cf. N_2O and air: 1.53 and 1.00 g/L and because of this it increases pulmonary airway resistance.
c. **False** – 0.14 compared with desflurane: 0.42. Note: xenon has the lowest blood gas (BG) partition coefficient of any inhalational anaesthetic agent.
d. **False** – it is very cardiovascular (CV) stable.
e. **True**.

151 Answers

a. **False** – $GABA_A$ receptors.
b. **True**.
c. **True**.
d. **False** – in clinical dosage they reduce electrical brain activity out of proportion to their effects on cellular homoeostasis.
e. **True** – enzyme induction is a hallmark of barbiturates.

152 Answers

a. **True** – propofol is 2,6 di-isopropyl phenol.
b. **False** – because it is a 'symmetrical' molecule. It has no asymmetric carbon atom(s).
c. **True**.
d. **True** – c. 7.0.
e. **True**.

153 Answers

a. **False** – cremophor EL (polyoxyethylene glycerol tri-ricinoleate) is no longer an additive because of its tendency to cause anaphylactic reactions.
b. **True** – in American preparations.
c. **True**.
d. **True**.
e. **False** – benzethonium is an additive in ketamine.

154 Answers

a. **True**.
b. **True**.
c. **False** – in lower dosage propofol is analgesic.
d. **True**.
e. **True**.

155 Answers

a. **True**.
b. **True**.
c. **True**.
d. **False** – ketamine acts by inhibition of the NMDA subtypes of glutamate receptors.
e. **True**.

156 Answers

a. **True**.
b. **True**.
c. **True** – a keto-enol tautomer. It is the enol form that renders it soluble.
d. **False** – it precipitates because of calcium in Hartmann's solution.
e. **False** – it owes its hypnotic effect to the substituted alkyl chains.

157 Answers

a. **True** – it produces a dissociative state but not true hypnosis.
b. **False** – although not a true bronchodilator, ketamine is nevertheless safe in asthmatics.
c. **True**.
d. **False** – ketamine can in fact increase jaw tone.
e. **True** – ketamine blocks re-uptake of noradrenaline.

158 Answers

a. **False** – although propofol has distinct analgesic activity, ketamine is the better analgesic.
b. **True** – thus it makes insertion of a laryngeal mask possible. Ketamine can increase jaw tone and sometimes produce laryngeal spasm.
c. **True** – ketamine has no true hypnotic properties.
d. **False** – ketamine produces a greater tachycardia because it has β-adrenergic agonist activity from blocking of re-uptake of catecholamines at their synaptic terminals.
e. **True** – propofol is metabolised by the CP 450 system to glucuronides and to corresponding quinol glucuronides and sulphates, which have no activity. Ketamine is broken down into norketamine, which has 30% of the activity of the parent compound.

159 Answers

a. **False** – adults more than children.
b. **True**.
c. **False**.
d. **False**.
e. **False**.

160 Answers

a. **False** – halothane is a substituted alkane; the others are substituted ethers.
b. **False** – all are chiral agents except sevoflurane.
c. **False** – halothane is the only one that contains a preservative, i.e. thymol 0.01%.
d. **False** – halothane is the only one so amenable, but all can be measured by infra-red analysis.
e. **True**.

161 Answer

Enflurane is the only one reputed to cause cerebral excitation.

162 Answers

a. **False** – its MW is 168. Sevoflurane has the highest: 200; halothane: 197; enflurane and isoflurane being isomers have the same MW: 184.
b. **True** – the three carbon monoxide-forming agents are desflurane, enflurane and isoflurane (in that order) because they each possess a $-CHF_2$ moiety.
c. **True** – having the lowest boiling point of all the inhalational agents (22.9°C), its vapour pressure at room temperature (21°C) is the highest (669 mmHg).
d. **True** – 6–7%.
e. **False** – lowest 0.02%.

163 Answers

a. **True**.
b. **True**.
c. **True** – bromochlorodifluruoethylene.
d. **False** – sevoflurane does not either.
e. **False** – enflurane has also been implicated.

164 Answers

a. **True** – it resides in the benzoic acid, which is an aromatic acid.
b. **False** – it depends on the amino acid fraction.
c. **False** – it is the aromatic radical that imparts potency.
d. **True**.
e. **False** – the laevorotatory forms are less toxic than the dextrorotatory forms.

165 Answers

a. **True** – with a typical pH of c. 8–9.
b. **True** – except for lignocaine and amethocaine, which are achiral.
c. **True** – they have a pH of c. 3.0–6.5.
d. **True** – except for cocaine and ropivacaine.
e. **True** – especially the amide-linked LAs.

166 Answers

a. **True** – because they are broken down by plasma esterases.
b. **True**.
c. **True**.
d. **True**.
e. **False** – amide LAs are bound to α_1-acid glycoprotein.

167 Answers

a. **False** – amethocaine is neither.
b. **True**.
c. **False** – it is an amide compound but not chiral.
d. **True**.
e. **True**.

168 Answers

a. **False** – it is obtained from *Erythroxylon coca*. Chondrodendron tomentosum is the plant from which curare is obtained.
b. **True** – all the others are synthetic agents.
c. **True** – it owes its vasoconstricting activity to this property.
d. **True** – same as **c**.
e. **False** – ropivacaine too has vasoconstricting activity.

169 Answers

a. **True**.
b. **True**.
c. **True** – by the process of de-alkylation.
d. **True**.
e. **False** – the metabolites released into the gut by biliary excretion are re-absorbed and then excreted in the urine.

170 Answers

a. **True**.
b. **True**.
c. **True** – about 50 times.
d. **True**.
e. **True**.

171 Answers

a. **True** – because it is cleared quickly from the blood by rapid tissue uptake.
b. **True**.
c. **False** – it causes little vasodilatation.
d. **True**.
e. **True**.

172 Answers

a. **True**.
b. **True**.
c. **True**.
d. **False** – because of lack of proven naloxone sensitivity.
e. **True**.

173 Answers

a. **True**.
b. **True**.
c. **True**.
d. **False** – it is reduced (see **c** above.) If adenylyl cyclase is inhibited, cAMP production must necessarily decrease.
e. **False** – neurotransmitter release is inhibited.

174 Answers

a. **True**.
b. **False** – leads to an anti-diuresis. Diuresis is caused by kappa receptor activation.
c. **True**.
d. **True**.
e. **True**.

175 Answers

a. **False** – morphine, codeine and thebaine are phenanthrene derivatives. Papaverine and noscapine are benzylisoquinoline derivatives.
b. **False** – relatively selective. In high doses it can interact with other types of opioid receptors.
c. **False** – it is good for nociceptive pain, but poor for neuropathic pain.
d. **False**.
e. **True** – morphine-6-glucuronide is at least twice as potent an analgesic as morphine.

176 Answers

a. **True**.
b. **False** – it is dose related. It is agonist/antagonist opioid analgesics, such as buprenorphine and nalbuphine, that suffer the ceiling effect.
c. **False** – except at very high dosage, the rate is usually diminished; the tidal volume usually increases.
d. **False** – hypoxia compounds the problem.
e. **True** – it almost always does.

177 Answers

a. **True**.
b. **True**.
c. **True** – 40–60% compared with 25% for morphine.
d. **True**.
e. **False** – higher renal excretion on acid diuresis because it is more dissociated in an acid medium.

178 Answers

a. It is an agonist/antagonist. Antagonist at μ receptors and an agonist at κ_1 and κ_3 receptors.
b. **True**.
c. **False** – see **a**.
d. **True**.
e. **False** – less prone.

179 Answers

a. **True**.
b. **True** – binds primarily to μ opioid receptors to produce its analgesic effect.
c. **False** – of the four stereo-isomers only the alpha racemate, propoxyphene, has analgesic activity, which resides in its dextro isomer, d-propoxyphene (dextropropoxyphene).
d. **False** – possesses only half to two-thirds the analgesic potency of codeine.
e. **True** – to norpropoxyphene, which accumulates following repeated dosage of propoxyphene.

180 Answers

a. **False** – act via $GABA_A$ receptors.
b. **True** – diazepam: 99%; midazolam: 94–97%; lorazepam: 85%.
c. **False**.
d. **True**.
e. **False**.

181 Answers

a. **False** – a highly negatively charged substance.
b. **True** – mast cells are the predominant site of heparin formation, but it is present to a lesser extent in basophils.
c. **False** – heparin has only a slight anticoagulant effect on its own. When combined with antithrombin III its effectiveness in removing thrombin is enhanced 100–1000-fold.
d. **True**.
e. **False** – protamine reversal of heparin is a chemical neutralisation.

182 Answers

a. **True**.
b. **False** – because its action is 'biological', not merely 'chemical'.
c. **False** – highly bound to plasma *albumin* up to 99%.
d. **False** – pharmacological competitive antagonism.
e. **True**.

183 Answers

a. **True** – a mucopolysaccharide present adsorbed on the inner surface of the vascular endothelium.
b. **True** – a protein bound to the vascular endothelium. It binds thrombin by: (i) removing thrombin; (ii) forming a complex with thrombin, which activates protein C, and which in turn inactivates Factor V and Factor VIII.
c. **True** – a plasma zymogen homologous to Factors II, VII, IX and X.
d. **True** – a 360,000 Da molecule that combines with coagulation factors.
e. **False** – plasminogen (also known as profibrinolysin) when activated to plasmin lyses fibrin.

184 Answers

a. **True** – it has three disulphide bonds; two of them are intersubunit in position, the third is intrasubunit.
b. **False** – MW: c. 5800; albumin: MW: 69,000.
c. **False** – is carried in the plasma as a free monomer.
d. **False** – insulin is an anabolic agent and therefore builds up proteins from amino acids, therefore urea levels fall.
e. **False** – insulin decreases, glucose increases the glucosyl valine adduct of Hb A1c.

185 **Answers**

a. **True**.
b. **True**.
c. **True**.
d. **True**.
e. **True**.

186 **Answers**

a. **False** – sulphonylurea.
b. **False** – sulphonylurea.
c. **False** – sulphonylurea.
d. **True**.
e. **False** – a thiazolidinedione derivative.

187 **Answers**

a. **False**.
b. **True**.
c. **True**.
d. **True**.
e. **False**.

188 **Answers**

a. **True**.
b. **True** – the adrenal medulla is equivalent to a sympathetic ganglion.
c. **True** – see above.
d. **True** – all ganglia, sympathetic and parasympathetic, are nicotinic ACh receptors.
e. **False** – sweat glands have postganglionic sympathetic terminals, but release acetycholine, so they have muscarinic receptors.

189 **Answers**

a. **False** – B type carboxylesterase.
b. **True**.
c. **True**.
d. **False** – undergoes carbamation.
e. **True**.

190 **Answers**

a. **True**.
b. **True**.
c. **False** – it cannot be used for TOF.
d. **False** – difficult to achieve.
e. **False** – the apparatus is bulky and heavy.

191 Answers

a. **True**.
b. **False** – the stimulus must have a square wave pattern.
c. **False** – the wave must be monophasic.
d. **True** – a higher current strength may lead to direct stimulation of the muscle.
e. **False** – must be less than 0.5 ms, preferably about 0.1–0.3 ms.

192 Answers

a. **True** – contrast that with non-depolarization block in which there is 'fade'.
b. **True**.
c. **True** – this is maintained, although reduced. cx. non-depolarising block where there is fade with tetanic stimulation.
d. **True** – occurs in Phase II block following large doses of depolarising relaxant.
e. **False** – anticholinesterases will extend the block.

193 Answers

a. **True**.
b. **True**.
c. **True**.
d. **False** – it is known to cause hyperkalaemia, especially in burn patients, but not hypokalaemia.
e. **True**.

194 Answers

a. **False** – it is an endogenous nucleoside.
b. **True** – specific G protein-coupled adenosine receptors.
c. **False** – its half-life is a few seconds.
d. **True** – by acting via A_2 (adenosine$_2$) receptors.
e. **False** – is taken up by most cells including cells of the endothelium and metabolised by adenosine deaminase to inosine.

195 Answers

a. **True**.
b. **True**.
c. **True**.
d. **True**.
e. **False** – smokers have a lower incidence of PONV than non-smokers.

196 Answers

a. **True**.

b. **True** – it is a chlorinated procainamide derivative.

c. **True**.

d. **True** – it has weak 5 HT$_3$ receptor antagonism, i.e. in higher dosage it produces those effects.

e. **False** – only 30% is excreted unchanged; the rest is excreted as sulphate and glucuronide.

197 Answers

a. **True**.

b. **True** – this drug has been withdrawn because of its propensity to cause prolonged QT interval.

c. **False**.

d. **False**.

e. **False**.

198 Answers

a. **False** – halothane is a racemic mixture of its (R) and (S) enantiomers, but they are anaesthetically equipotent. (Their difference lies in the fact that the (R) isomer produces significantly greater amounts of TFA-protein adducts in the liver than the (S) isomer.)

b. **False** – both ketamine isomers are anaesthetic and analgesic but the (S) isomer) is about three times as potent as the (R) isomer.

c. **True** – the (S) form is the anti-hypertensive and anti-anginal agent. The (R) form lacks cardiovascular activity but is useful in the treatment of hypothyroidism.

d. **True** – the (R) and (S) enantiomers are both equally active hypnotics, but the (S) isomer produces metabolites that are teratogenic.

e. **False** – both forms are calcium channel blockers, but (S) verapamil is 10–20 times more potent as an anti-arrhythmic, anti-hypertensive and anti-anginal agent than the (R) form.

199 Answers

a. **False** – it is an ester of acetic acid.

b. **False** – it is its acetyl moiety that is the active radical that inhibits cyclo-oxygenase.

c. **False** – c. 80–90% bound to plasma proteins.

d. **False** – excreted as (a) free salicylic acid (10%), (b) salicyluric acid (75%), (c) glucuronides (5%).

e. **False** – aspirin is not recognised as being an addictive drug.

200 Answers

a. **True** – because of the risk of Reye's syndrome (described 1963), a fulminant encephalopathy and acute hepatic dysfunction usually following a viral infection, varicella or 'flu' and associated with the use of aspirin during the viral illness.
b. **True**.
c. **False**.
d. **True** – because of the likelihood of haemolysis.
e. **False** – it is best avoided in *nasal* polyposis.

201 Answers

a. **False**.
b. **True**.
c. **True**.
d. **True**.
e. **True**.

Note: the degree of ionisation of a drug is dependent on the proximity of the drug's pKa to the environmental pH. The nearer they are to each other, the lower the degree of ionisation. The gastric luminal pH is c. 2 and therefore aspirin in the stomach is mainly in un-ionised form. The pH of the other sites are as follows: gastric epithelial cell: c. 7.4; lower small intestine: 7.6; plasma: 7.4.

202 Answers

a. **False**.
b. **True** – phenacetin, which is no longer used, exerts its effects at least partly as paracetamol.
c. **False** – it has no anti-inflammatory properties.
d. **False** – in large doses has weakly inhibitory effects on cyclo-oxygenase.
e. **False** – 60% as the glucuronide; 35% as the sulphate; 3% combined with cysteine.

203 Answers

a. **True** – apart from its effect on platelet adhesiveness, aspirin can also cause a hypoprothrombinaemia.
b. **False**.
c. **True**.
d. **True** – may prolong and enhance the action of warfarin.
e. **True**.

204   Answers

a. **True**.
b. **False** – aspirin is more likely to cause haemolysis, especially in persons with glucose-6-phosphate dehydrogenase deficiency.
c. **True** – indeed methaemoglobinaemia is a common side effect in AIDS patients as a side effect of treatment with primaquine (and dapsone).
d. **False** – sulphaemoglobinaemia is the side effect produced by phenacetin.
e. **True** – see **c**. Dapsone can also cause sulphaemoglobinaemia.

205   Answers

a. **True** – for animals it is the ratio LD_{50}/ED_{50}, i.e. the dose that is lethal in 50% of animals (LD_{50}) divided by the dose that has the desired effect in 50% of animals (ED_{50}).
b. **False** – cardiac index is the cardiac output per square metre of body surface area: litres per minute per metre^2.
c. **False** – body mass index: weight in kg/height in m^2. It was named after Lambert Adolphe Jacques Quetelet (1796–1874), Belgian statistician and sociologist.
d. **True** – degree of substitution of the OH groups of the anhydroglucose moieties of amylopectin with hydroxyethyl groups in hetastarch preparations.
e. **True** – the ratio of the speed of light in one medium to that in an adjacent medium (important in fibreoptic transmission of light).

206   Answer

a. **False** – the slope of the 'Hill plot', i.e. the log–dose response curve. The response as a percentage of maximum response per unit log dose of drug.

b. **False** – Faraday constant: number of coulombs of electrical energy per gram equivalent of element: 9.65×10^4 coulombs per gram equivalent.

c. **True** – Reynolds' number $= v\rho d/\eta$,

Where v: linear velocity of fluid; ρ: fluid density; d: tube diameter; η: viscosity of fluid. The dimensions of the various factors cancel out each other, rendering Reynolds' number dimensionless.

d. **True** – the reflection coefficient s is the ratio of the observed colloid osmotic pressure difference to the theoretical colloid osmotic pressure difference across a membrane which is deemed impermeable to colloids but nevertheless permits some colloid 'leak' across it. The value of s ranges from 0 to 1. When s is zero the moving water carries the colloid solute with it and therefore the colloid exerts no osmotic pressure at all. When s is 1, the barrier completely excludes the solute colloid, which then exerts its full colloid osmotic pressure.

e. **True** – also known as 'relative permittivity'. It is the extent to which a capacitor 'permits' the passage of electric current through its 'dielectric', i.e. the material intervening between the two plates of the capacitor, which may even be air, relative to that permitted by a vacuum. Therefore it is a ratio and thus dimensionless.

207   Answers

a. **True**.
b. **True**.
c. **True**.
d. **True**.
e. **False**.

208   Answers

a. **False** – the ampere is a unit of 'rating', i.e. a phenomenon – in this case the flow of current energy (coulombs)-per unit time (seconds).

b. **False** – lumen is candela per steradian per second. The corresponding 'intensity' unit is 'lux', which is 'lumen per square metre'.

c. **True** – newtons per square metre.

d. **False** – the watt is a 'rating', i.e. a phenomenon – in this case energy (joules) – per unit time (seconds).

e. **False** – weber is the unit of magnetic flux. The corresponding 'intensity' unit is the tesla, which is 'magnetic flux density' and is 'webers per square metre'.

209 Answers

a. **True** – I torr is almost the same as I mmHg.
b. **True**.
c. **False** – 100,000 newtons per square metre.
d. 1,000,000 dynes per square centimetre.
e. **True**.

210 Answers

a. **True** – because osmolarity is the number of osmoles of solute per *litre* of solution, i.e. per unit *volume*, and volume is temperature dependent. cx. 'osmolality', which is the number of osmoles of solute per *kilogram* of solvent (water). This is independent of temperature, because mass is not temperature dependent.
b. **False** – see **a**.
c. **True** – because the solubility of an agent in blood is temperature dependent.
d. **True** – see **c**.
e. **False**.

211 Answers

a. **True** – this is Boyle's law.
b. **True**.
c. **True**.
d. **False** – the graph is that of an accelerating growth exponential.
e. **False** – the graph is a straight line.

Note: where the relationship between two entities takes the form:

$A \alpha \dfrac{1}{B}$ the graphic depiction is that of a rectangular hyperbola.

212 Answers

a. **True**.
b. **True**.
c. **True**.
d. **False** – this is not part of the definition of an ideal gas.
e. **False** – will render an 'ideal gas' non-ideal and thus the definition of an 'ideal gas' invalid.

213 Answers

a. **True** – i.e. there are no internal frictional forces in the fluid, i.e. the fluid has no viscosity.
b. **False** – a fluid whose behaviour conforms to the Hagen–Poiseuille law is a 'newtonian' fluid.
c. **False** – a thixotropic fluid is one whose shear rate varies with flow rate (blood is a thixotropic fluid), i.e. it must have a changing viscosity and therefore it is a 'non-newtonian' fluid.
d. **False**.
e. **False**.

214 Answers

a. **True** – the light beam does not diverge.
b. **True** – the waves are all in phase.
c. **False** – cavitation is a property of ultrasonic waves.
d. **False** – precession is a property of magnetic resonance imaging (MRI).
e. **True** – there is a higher percentage of activated atoms in the laser substrate compared with that of quiescent atoms. The atom population has been 'inverted'.

215 Answers

a. **True**.
b. **True**.
c. **True**.
d. **True**.
e. **True**.

216 Answers

a. **True**.
b. **True** – cylinders for use in the MRI scanner room are made of aluminium.
c. **False** – a black body and white shoulders.
d. **False** – filling ratios apply only to cylinders that contain the agent in both liquid and gaseous form.
e. **False** – the positions are 2 and 5.

217 Answers

a. **True**.
b. **False** – 1 and 5.
c. **False** – 1 and 6.
d. **True**.
e. **True**.

218 Answers

a. **False** – apart from cylinder size, the absence of a pin index outlet precludes attachment of a size F oxygen cylinder to an anaesthetic machine.

b. **False** – CO_2 cylinders C, D and E can all be coupled to the pin index attachment of an anaesthetic machine that has provision for administration of CO_2.

c. **False** – full cyclopropane cylinders have a pressure of only 7 atmospheres and therefore do not require a pressure regulator in the gas pathway.

d. **False** – because while their 'downstream' pressure is the same, i.e. 4 bar, their 'upstream' pressures are different: 137 bar for oxygen; c.45–50 bar for nitrous oxide.

e. **False** – anaesthetic machine air: 400 kPa; surgical drill air: 700 kPa.

219 Answers

a. **True** – mass spectrometry can be used to assay any gas.

b. **False** – IR analysis requires the presence of at least two dissimilar atoms in the molecule of the gas to be analysed.

c. **True** – Raman scattering is applicable provided the molecules are divalent.

d. **True** – a gas is paramagnetic, and therefore amenable to paramagnetic analysis, provided its atoms or molecules have unpaired electrons. Oxygen is one such gas.

e. **True** – pyrogallol absorbs oxygen and therefore the method can be used for measuring oxygen, but it is not used today.

220 Answers

a. **True** – infra-red analysis can be used to measure any gas that has two or more dissimilar elements.

b. **False** – to be measurable by Raman scattering a gas must have molecules that are at least diatomic.

c. **True** – all halogenated inhalational agents can be measured by the piezo-electric crystal method.

d. **True** – in fact halothane was estimated in the past by this method.

e. **True** – mass spectrometry can be used to estimate any gas.

221 Answers

a. **True**.

b. **False** – they must be different. In the Clark electrode the anode is Ag/AgCl and the cathode is platinum.

c. **False** – at the cathode.

d. **True** – it involves reaction between O_2 and water as follows:

$$O_2 + 4e + 2 H_2O = 4(OH)^-$$

e. **False** – the temperature needs to be kept at a fixed level.

222 Answers

a. **False** – Mapleson C. It can be made into a 'D' by the incorporation of a length of corrugated hose between the Y connection and the valve–bag unit.

b. **False** – Less efficient. The test of 'efficiency' is determined by the ratio of the fresh gas flow rate (sufficient to maintain near-normocapnia) and the patient's minute ventilation. The lower the ratio the more efficient the attachment.

c. **False** – efferent limb.

d. **True** – but it would be wasteful of gases.

e. **False** – because, among other things, the resistance through the adjustable pressure-limiting valve (APL) valve would be too high and the apparatus dead space would be too large.

223 Answers

a. **True**.

b. **False** – essentially exhaled gases.

c. **True** – behaves essentially as the Magill.

d. **True** – same behaviour as in **c**.

e. **False** – a mixture of fresh gases and exhaled gases.

224 Answers

a. **False**.

b. **False**.

c. **False**.

d. **True**.

e. **False**.

Note: the 'efficiency' of a breathing attachment is defined by determining the lowest fresh gas flow rate required (relative to the patient's minute volume) that is capable of maintaining near-normocapnia. By this criterion the parallel Lack is considered the best, followed by the Magill and then the Lack co-axial attachments. The Bain and Ayre's T-piece attachments are regarded as the 'worst'.

225 Answers

a. **True**.

b. **True**.

c. **False** – wetness will make the soda lime less granular and therefore more compact.

d. **False**.

e. **False**.

226 Answers

a. **True** – also known as phosgene, carbonyl chloride was a by-product of reaction between trichloroethylene (now no longer used) and soda lime.

b. **False** – methane accumulates because of release from the patient, not from reaction between soda lime and inhalational agents.

c. **False** – very minute amounts of nitrogen dioxide may be a contaminant present in N_2O cylinders, but in the breathing attachment not as a result of reaction between soda lime and inhaled N_2O.

d. **True** – it is 'Compound A', produced as a reaction between sevoflurane and soda lime.

e. **True** – a halothane breakdown product.

227 Answers

a. **True**.

b. **False**.

c. **True**.

d. **False** – it may make it more marked.

e. **False** – if there is less liquid agent, then there is a larger air space above it, which will allow for more carrier gas to 'backtrack' into the vaporising chamber, thereby making the pumping effect even more marked.

228 Answers

a. **True**.

b. **True**.

c. **True**.

d. **True**.

e. **True**.

229 Answers

a. **True**.

b. **True**.

c. **True**.

d. **True**.

e. **True**.

230 Answers

a. **True**.

b. **False**.

c. **True**.

d. **True**.

e. **False** – delivers a constant 'volumes per cent' of vapour.

231 Answers

a. **False** – the gas pressure beyond the 'needle valve' of the flowmeter unit is about 30–40 kPa gauge pressure.
b. **True**.
c. **True**.
d. **False** – the driving energy is provided by the very gases that are used to fill the patients' lungs and these come up the flowmeter unit and then along the back bar. See **a**.
e. **True** – was in common use before the advent of automatic sphygmomanometers.

232 Answers

a. **True**.
b. **False** – they need to be rendered antistatic to prevent the bobbins sticking to the sidewall of the tube.
c. **False**.
d. **True** – in the bottom half of the tube, viscosity; in the top half, density.
e. **False** – flowmeter tubes are non-interchangeable for reasons of cross-sectional area, bobbin size etc., and not for reasons of height alone.

233 Answers

a. **True**.
b. **True** – so as to match the patient's peak inspiratory flow rate.
c. **True** – the ISO regulations.
d. **False**.
e. **False** – but it will necessarily reduce the flow rate in the rotameter tube.

234 Answers

a. **True** – necessary for the chemical reactions involved in CO_2 absorption and also to minimise the formation of carbon monoxide.
b. **True** – NaOH is a catalyst that hastens the combination of CO_2 with soda lime.
c. **True** – $Ca(OH)_2$ is the definitive reactant for CO_2 absorption.
d. **False** – KOH is no longer necessary and indeed ought to be avoided so as to minimise the chances of CO generation.
e. **True** – granularity: (i) increases the surface area for CO_2 absorption; and (ii) minimises obstruction to gas flow through the soda lime.

235 Answers

a. **True**.
b. **True**.
c. **True** – so as to minimise the current density and thereby eliminate the risk of diathermy burn.
d. **True**.
e. **False** – the aim is to eliminate any air between probe and skin surface and thereby minimise acoustic mismatch.

236 Answers

a. **True** – about 1.5–3.5 MHz.
b. **True** – about 3.5 MHz.
c. **True** – the frequency is c. 10^{12} Hz.
d. **False** – c. 50,000 Hz
e. **True** – the frequency is c. 10^{12} Hz.

237 Answers

a. **False** – DC electricity can cause VF but requires about 20–30% more current energy for the purpose.
b. **False** – laser pointers, for instance, are energised by dry cell batteries, which are DC.
c. **True** – AC electricity has been used in the past but not very effectively.
d. To produce an US beam of say 3 MHz frequency an AC supply at the same frequency is required.
e. **False** – 'cautery,' as opposed to 'diathermy', is usually effected by using an appliance that produces DC electricity of low voltage (c. 10–20 V).

238 Answers

a. **True**.
b. **False** – the symbol is a 'box within a box'. It is Class I equipment that has no symbol.
c. **True** – it is 'safety extra low voltage' (SELV) equipment: the power may be from a battery or it may be a mains voltage suitably stepped down by means of a transformer.
d. **True** – but if the earth cable is disconnected then the voltage of the appliance may be such as to cause electrocution.
e. **True** – the International Electrotechnical Commission (IEC) mandates that the permitted leakage current for CF equipment is 50 μA, for BF equipment is 500 μA.

239 Answers

a. True – because the voltage is alternating, it never reaches steady-state conditions, and therefore in accordance with Ohm's law, neither can the current.

b. True.

c. False – the reactance (i.e. the opposition to current flow) in an inductor is directly proportional to the rate of change of voltage. In the case of a capacitor such opposition is inversely proportional to frequency of alternation of current.

d. False – the opposition to current flow is called 'reactance', which is one form of 'impedance'. Like resistance, it is measured in ohms. The mho is the reciprocal of ohms and therefore is the unit of electrical conductance. It has now been replaced by the 'siemens', after Karl William (later Sir Charles William) Siemens, who became a naturalised British subject.

e. True – reactance is the opposition to current flow in an AC circuit which contains a capacitor and/or inductor.

240 Answers

a. False – an 'isolated' unit and an 'REM' plate serve two different and unrelated functions. 'Isolation' from earth is to prevent electrocution of the patient as a result of 'leakage currents'. An REM plate helps check the degree of contact between diathermy plate and skin, and thereby warns of increased current density and thus minimises a skin burn under the plate.

b. True – see **a** above.

c. False – a 'return electrode' plate is necessary to provide monopolar mode, which is necessary for cutting diathermy, but it need not be an 'REM' plate.

d. True – no (return electrode) plate, be it REM plate or other, is necessary when using the bipolar mode.

e. False – a need for a diathermy plate, REM or otherwise, is not removed merely because the switch is hand operated.

241 Answers

a. True.

b. True – it is this that gives O_2 its paramagnetic property and also makes it a 'diradical'.

c. True – but not to the same extent as ozone.

d. True – mass spectrometry can analyse any gas.

e. True.

242 Answers

a. False.

b. True – at pressures of 30 atmospheres nitrogen is a narcotic.

c. False – the solubility coefficient (ml per litre of solvent per 1 atmosphere 100 kPa pressure). For N_2 it is c. 12 ml; for O_2 it is about 24 ml.

d. False – it is about 5–6 times more soluble in fat than in water.

e. True – the alveolar pN_2 is c. 80 kPa, at which each litre of body water will have about 9.6 ml of nitrogen (see *solubility coefficient* under **c.**). The solubility of N_2 in fat is about 5–6 times that in water. On this basis the total amount of nitrogen present *dissolved* in body tissues is about 1 L. The total lung capacity is about 5–6 L, therefore at an alveolar p N_2 of c. 80 kPa the total volume of nitrogen is c. 4–5 L.

243 Answers

a. False – it constitutes about 0.03% of atmospheric air.

b. True – because size C, D and E carbon dioxide cylinders all have pin index outlets.

c. False – a full CO_2 cylinder has a pressure of c. 50 bar, a full O_2 cylinder c. 137 bar.

d. False – it is an exothermic reaction.

e. False – unlike the combination of CO_2 with water to form bicarbonate, the formation of carbaminohaemoglobin is not enzyme dependent.

244 Answers

a. False – helium has a higher viscosity than nitrogen: 0.0198 mPa s, compared with 0.0179 for nitrogen (both measured at 25°C).

b. False – hydrogen is lighter than helium.

c. False – in lower airway obstruction it is the viscosity of the gas that is the material factor, therefore helium is not of any benefit.

d. False – uniatomic gases cannot be measured by Raman scattering.

e. True – therefore it is used as a supercoolant in the MRI scanner.

245 Answers

a. False – is obtained by heating ammonium nitrate: $NH_4NO_3 \rightarrow N_2O + 2H_2O$.

b. True – several times sweeter than sucrose.

c. True – in fact at a temperature of c. 400°C nitrous oxide can explode.

d. False – by selectively inhibiting glutamate-stimulated currents mediated by NMDA receptors.

e. False – small amounts diffuse through the skin.

a. **False** – it will not, because the contents are partly liquid.
b. **True** – because the liquid N_2O will take up its latent heat of vaporisation from the cylinder contents and ambient air, which may cause the temperature to fall so low as to lead to frost formation.
c. **True**.
d. **True** – for the same reason as in **b**, any water inside the cylinder will freeze and clog the outlet port.
e. **False**.

247   Answers

Principle: provided the agent is solely in gaseous form the reading accurately reflects the number of moles of the agent in it. This holds because of the Universal Gas Equation PV = nRT. In the case of a cylinder, V (internal volume of the cylinder), R and T are constants. Therefore Pα n, the number of moles of the gas.

a. **True**.
b. **False**.
c. **True**.
d. **False**.
e. **True**.

248   Answers

a. **True** – 'semi-conductor': a material (including some solids as silicon and germanium) whose (feeble) electrical conductivity is neither metallic (moving electrons) nor electrolytic (moving ions).
b. **False** – semi-conductors (and insulators) have a negative temperature coefficient, i.e. their resistance decreases with a rise in temperature. cx. metals, which have a positive temperature coefficient.
c. **False** – measures resistance change. See **b**.
d. **True** – resistance varies about 4% per degree Celsius and can be measured to an accuracy of c. 0.01°C.
e. **True**.

249   Answers

a. **True** – covalent bonds are the strongest of chemical bonds.
b. **True** – hydrogen bonds are responsible for many of the physical properties of water.
c. **True**.
d. **True**.
e. **False** – all bonds in methane are non-polar covalent in nature, which accounts for the extreme stability of methane.

250 Answers

a. **False** – weak intermolecular forces.
b. **False** – they are 'non-bonding' attractions.
c. **True**.
d. **True**.
e. **False** – the relationship: the product of the magnitude of the forces is inversely proportional to the seventh power of the distance separating them.

251 Answers

a. **False**.
b. **True** – aspirin acetylates the serine residue of cyclo-oxygenase.
c. **False**.
d. **True**.
e. **False**.

252 Answers

a. **True**.
b. **False** – dynamic isomerism is *keto-enol tautomerism*, a form of structural isomerism. *cis-trans* isomerism is a form of stereo-isomerism.
c. **False** – in straight chain compounds a double bond is an essential pre-requisite for *cis-trans* isomerism, but the phenomenon can also be present in compounds with a ring structure, even without the presence of double bonds.
d. **True** – cell membrane fatty acids are invariably unsaturated fatty acids and therefore have carbon–carbon double bonds and are usually of the *cis* form.
e. **True** – light is detected when photons of light reach the retina and change *cis*-retinal to *trans*-retinal, a change which is essential for generation of the nerve impulse that is to be transmitted along the optic nerve to the brain.

253 Answers

a. **True**.
b. **False** – they usually result from homolytic fission of covalent bonds. In heterolytic fission of a covalent bond both electrons end on one atom. In homolytic fission each atom ends up with one (unpaired) electron.
c. **True** – because in the case of oxygen, fission leads to both electrons ending as unpaired electrons on one atom of the molecule.
d. **True**.
e. **False** – they are secondary pollutants, which are the free radicals formed when the primary pollutants are acted upon by sunlight.

254   Answers

a. **True**.
b. **True**.
c. **True**.
d. **True**.
e. **True**.

255   Answers

a. **True** – it is the same as vitamin E.
b. **True** – it is vitamin A.
c. **False**.
d. **False**.
e. **False**.

256   Answers

a. **False** – radiation accounts for about 40–50% of the total heat loss from the body.
b. **False** – it is in the form of infra-red radiations.
c. **True** – radiation is the only form of heat loss that can occur through a vacuum, which explains why the sun's radiant energy can appear on earth, having travelled a distance of 93 million miles mostly through empty space.
d. **False** – heat loss through evaporation (respiration and perspiration) is the only mode that can occur against a temperature gradient.
e. **False** – no matter their skin complexion, all humans behave as 'black bodies', i.e. they tend to absorb (almost) all EMRs incident on them and emit all such radiations, (in addition to emitting the heat radiations produced as a result of metabolic processes).

257   Answers

a. **True**.
b. **False** – they are more effective with increasing chain length (i.e. number of carbon atoms) up to about 5–8. Beyond that their efficacy wanes.
c. **False** – straight-chain alcohols are more effective than isoforms and for that reason tertiary alcohols are the least effective.
d. **False** – alcohols are most effective as sterilants at a concentration of between 60 and 80%.
e. **True**.

258 Answers

a. **False**.
b. **False** – povidone iodine can be sporicidal but only on long exposure.
c. **True**.
d. **True**.
e. **False**.

259 Answers

a. **True**.
b. **True**.
c. **True**.
d. **False** – xenon too undergoes no known biotransformation.
e. **True**.

260 Answers

a. **True** – during quiet spontaneous ventilation the intrapleural pressure is always 'negative', i.e. subatmospheric.
b. **True** – up to c. -3 cm H_2O.
c. **True** – 1.5 to $-$ 15 mmHg.
d. **True** – c. -4 to -6 mmHg.
e. **True** – c. -4 to -6 mmHg.

Practice paper I

Anatomy

1.1 The following skull foramina convey cranial nerves:

a. Foramina of cribriform plate of ethmoid.
b. Foramen rotundum.
c. Foramen spinosum.
d. Jugular foramen.
e. Foramen lacerum.

1.2 The following intracranial veins are paired structures:

a. Basilar sinus.
b. Sigmoid sinus.
c. Occipital sinus.
d. Transverse sinus.
e. Posterior cavernous sinus.

1.3 When performing a lumbar puncture the needle must necessarily penetrate the following structures:

a. Superficial fascia.
b. Supraspinous ligament.
c. Interspinous ligament.
d. Ligamentum denticulatum.
e. Piamater.

1.4 The vagus nerves:

a. Both leave the cranium via the foramen magnum.
b. Both give rise to their respective recurrent laryngeal branches at the level of the Angle of Louis.
c. Each possesses a 'superior' and an 'inferior' sensory ganglion.
d. Both contribute in equal measure to the anterior vagal trunk of the stomach.
e. Both equally contribute a supply to the coeliac plexus.

1.5   **In the case of the diaphragm:**

   a. Its left and right crura arise from the same lumbar vertebrae.

   b. Both its sensory and motor nerve supplies are solely from the phrenic nerves.

   c. Its oesophageal opening is more anterior than its caval opening.

   d. Its aortic opening transmits just the aorta alone.

   e. Its caval opening is at the level of the 12th thoracic vertebra.

Physiology

1.6 The Na⁺–K⁺–ATPase pump:

a. Is a homodimer.
b. Is a symport system.
c. Has a coupling ratio of $Na^+ - K^+ = 2 - 3$.
d. Has faster rates of transmembranal Na^+ and K^+ movements than those through Na^+ and K^+ ion channels.
e. Undergoes inhibition as part of the necessary pharmacological activity of cardiac glycosides.

1.7 Facilitated diffusion:

a. Is a carrier-mediated transport process.
b. Requires an input of extraneous energy.
c. Is a saturable process.
d. Is temperature dependent.
e. Is exemplified by amino acid absorption in the renal tubule.

1.8 The following processes are usually enzyme dependent:

a. Combination of CO_2 with haemoglobin to form carbaminohaemoglobin.
b. Hydration of CO_2 in the plasma to form H_2CO_3.
c. Biotransformation of atracurium.
d. Production of nitric oxide.
e. Formation of pyruvate in the Embden–Meyerhof pathway.

1.9 Haemoglobin:

a. Is a tetrameric protein.
b. Possesses the attribute of 'allosterism'.
c. In its HbA form has a higher P_{50} than haemoglobin F.
d. Has 2,3 diphosphoglycerate better bound to it than to haemoglobin F.
e. When oxygenated, changes its structure from the 'T' 'taut' form to the 'R' 'relaxed' form.

1.10 The following are factors or features associated with red cell haemoglobin activity:

a. Hufner constant.
b. Valtis–Kennedy effect.
c. Fink phenomenon.
d. Fahraeus–Lindqvist effect.
e. Rapaport–Luebering shunt.

1.11 The binding of oxygen to haemoglobin:

a. Is an allosteric phenomenon.
b. Is one of oxidation.
c. Occurs at the fifth coordination position of the Fe^{2+} ion.
d. Makes the iron ion smaller.
e. Makes the iron ion more magnetic.

1.12 In the case of carbonic anhydrase:

a. It is type II carbonic anhydrase that is found in red cells.
b. It contains zinc as an essential ingredient in its structure.
c. It is maximally active at high pH.
d. It is a histidine molecule that is the group responsible for its hydrating activity.
e. It can hydrate CO_2 more than a million times faster than the 'spontaneous' reaction.

1.13 In the alimentary tract:

a. Tight junctions get progressively 'tighter' down the alimentary canal.
b. The small intestinal contents are usually isotonic with plasma.
c. Na^+ is absorbed along the entire length of the intestine.
d. More water is absorbed in the ileum than in the jejunum.
e. K^+ absorption is essentially a passive process.

1.14 The following are of the same magnitude in the cerebrospinal fluid as in the plasma:

a. Osmolarity.
b. Sodium concentration.
c. Potassium concentration.
d. Chloride concentration.
e. Glucose concentration.

1.15 During normal quiet spontaneous ventilation:

a. Chest expansion is solely dependent on diaphragmatic contraction.
b. The intrapleural pressure is always subatmospheric.
c. The energy expenditure is no more than about 5% of the body's basal energy usage.
d. Compliance work is the predominant reason for energy expenditure.
e. Expiration is essentially an active process.

1.16 During normal quiet spontaneous ventilation the following increase from top to bottom of the lung:

    a. The negativity of the intrapleural space.
    b. Pulmonary ventilation.
    c. Pulmonary blood flow.
    d. V/Q ratio.
    e. Pulmonary capillary pressure.

1.17 Surfactant:

    a. Is 100% phospholipids.
    b. Is formed by Type I cells of the alveoli.
    c. Has an alveolar half-life of about 7–10 days.
    d. Possesses antioxidant properties.
    e. Helps prevent pulmonary oedema.

1.18 The FEV_1 (forced expiratory volume in 1 second):

    a. Is the volume of air exhaled in 1 second starting immediately after a normal inspiration.
    b. Can be determined by simple bell spirometry.
    c. Is normally less than 50% of a forced vital capacity.
    d. Is less informative of lung dysfunction than is a FEV_2 or a FEV_3.
    e. As a ratio of the FVC (i.e. FEV_1/FVC) is higher in an obstructive pattern of breathing than in a restrictive pattern.

1.19 Hypoxic pulmonary vasoconstriction:

    a. Is a phenomenon present in all mammalian species.
    b. Occurs uniformly in all the segments of the pulmonary vasculature.
    c. Is mediated via centrally activated neural reflexes.
    d. Can proceed in the absence of intact endothelium.
    e. Is aggravated by hypocapnia.

1.20 The 'carotid body':

    a. Is a 'fast-responding' monitor of pO_2 and pCO_2 of arterial blood.
    b. Has the highest rate of perfusion of any organ in the body.
    c. Plays a greater role than the aortic bodies in blood gas homeostasis.
    d. Undergoes hypertrophy and hyperplasia under conditions of chronic hypoxia.
    e. Depends for its chemoreceptor function on its 'Type II' cells.

1.21 Concerning the autonomic nerve supply of the heart:

a. Its sympathetic component arises from thoracic spinal segments 4–8.
b. Under resting conditions the heart is under sympathetic domination.
c. The parasympathetic supply is essentially confined to the atria and their structures.
d. The atrioventricular node receives its parasympathetic supply from the right vagus nerve.
e. The sympathetic supply is solely of the β-adrenergic type.

1.22 Cardiac action potentials of the fast type occur in the:

a. Sinoatrial node.
b. Atrioventricular node.
c. Purkinje conduction system.
d. Atrial myocardium.
e. Ventricular myocardium.

1.23 Compared with an action potential of a ventricular myocardial cell, the action potential of the sino-atrial node:

a. Is less negative.
b. Has a steeper upstroke.
c. Has an absent plateau phase.
d. Has a faster depolarisation phase.
e. Is not affected by tetrodotoxin.

1.24 The following are reflexes relating to cardiac activity:

a. Bainbridge reflex.
b. Bezold–Jarisch reflex.
c. Brewer–Luckhardt reflex.
d. Cushing reflex.
e. Hering–Breuer reflex.

1.25 In the case of the heart:

a. It has the highest possible uptake of oxygen per unit mass of any organ.
b. Its venous blood oxygen saturation is normally lower than that of the brain.
c. At the end of diastole its atria contain more blood than its ventricles.
d. It is almost entirely dependent on glucose as its metabolic substrate.
e. It is essentially dependent on aerobic metabolism for its energy supply.

1.26 When measuring blood pressure with a mercury sphygmomanometer, a falsely higher systolic reading is more likely to be obtained if:

    a. A narrower cuff is used.
    b. If the cuff were to be applied over clothing.
    c. If the cuff were to be loosely applied to the arm.
    d. If cuff deflation was carried out more slowly.
    e. If the position of the zero reference point on the manometer was below heart level.

1.27 In the case of the arterial circulation in the recumbent subject:

    a. The systolic pressure is lower in the femoral artery than in the ascending aorta.
    b. The diastolic pressure remains more or less the same at all points in the arterial vasculature.
    c. The mean pressure decreases with increasing distance from the heart.
    d. The pulse waveform flattens as it moves down the arterial tree.
    e. The mean aortic pressure is lower than the mean left ventricular pressure.

1.28 Concerning the pulmonary veins:

    a. They are virtually inelastic.
    b. They have no valves.
    c. They account for about one-fifth to one-third of the pulmonary vascular resistance.
    d. They contain about 50% of the pulmonary blood volume.
    e. The blood flow in them is pulsatile.

1.29 Cerebral ischaemic injury:

    a. Is followed by a rise in intracellular Na^+.
    b. Is accompanied by release of large amounts of glutamate.
    c. Is worsened by a rise in cerebral perfusion pressure.
    d. Is associated with release of arachidonic acid from cell membranes.
    e. Leads to oxidative injury to cellular DNA.

1.30 The following anaesthetic agents are regarded as providing protection after cerebral injury:

    a. Thiopentone.
    b. Isoflurane.
    c. Propofol.
    d. Desflurane.
    e. Etomidate.

1.31 The liver:

a. Receives approximately equal blood flows from the hepatic artery and portal vein.
b. Extracts approximately equal volumes of oxygen per minute from hepatic artery blood and portal vein blood.
c. Contains approximately equal volumes of blood in its arteries, capillaries and veins.
d. Normally contains sufficient glycogen stores to provide energy during starvation for about 7 days.
e. Plays little or no role in erythropoiesis in the adult.

1.32 The following act as chelating agents in the situations referred to:

a. Edetate in blood sample bottles for full blood count.
b. Penicillamine in promoting urinary excretion of heavy metals.
c. Protamine sulphate in the reversal of heparin.
d. Desferrioxamine in iron binding in thalassaemia.
e. Edrophonium when inactivating acetylcholinesterase.

1.33 Brown adipose tissue:

a. Is labelled 'brown' because of its natural brown appearance in vivo.
b. Is only present after birth.
c. Is generally found in relation to large blood vessels.
d. Is under β-adrenergic control.
e. Contains thermogenin

1.34 Water:

a. Attracts and forms hydrogen bonds between its molecules.
b. Is self-ionised only to a very slight degree.
c. Has a high boiling point among common liquids.
d. Has a high surface tension.
e. Has a high dielectric constant.

1.35 When carbon dioxide is carried in the blood:

a. It is carried in the plasma primarily as carbonic acid.
b. It forms carbaminohaemoglobin by combining with the haem moiety of haemoglobin.
c. As a carbamate component it is present in the plasma.
d. The acidity it induces is buffered by means of the globin moieties of haemoglobin.
e. More than 50% of it is carried as plasma bicarbonate.

1.36. **Alcohol:**

a. Is a water-soluble substance.
b. Has a specific density higher than that of water.
c. Undergoes greater absorption in the stomach than the small intestine.
d. Has a volume of distribution greater than the plasma volume.
e. Readily enters the fetus through the placenta.

1.37 **Of the commonly used IV crystalloid solutions (Hartmann's solution, N-saline, 5% glucose and glucose-saline):**

a. The pH of glucose-saline is nearest that of the plasma.
b. N-saline is the most acidic.
c. Hartmann's solution has bicarbonate as a buffer.
d. Only 5% glucose has 'free water'.
e. All of them have an osmolarity less than that of the plasma.

1.38 **The following are safely usable as peritoneal insufflating gases for laparoscopy provided no diathermy or laser is used:**

a. Carbon dioxide.
b. Oxygen.
c. Nitrogen.
d. Nitrous oxide.
e. Helium.

1.39 **In the autonomic nervous system:**

a. Muscarinic receptor sites are present in parasympathetic ganglia.
b. A nicotinic effect is that which occurs exclusively at somatic motor nerve endings.
c. A muscarinic effect is by definition one that can be blocked by atropine.
d. Some nicotinic effects can be blocked with phenoxybenzamine.
e. Responses to nicotinic agonists are slower than those to muscarinic agonists.

1.40 **Concerning the enteric nervous system:**

a. It contains as many nerve cells as does the spinal cord.
b. It has greater local autonomy than the other divisions of the autonomic nervous system.
c. It has no sensory component.
d. Its principal excitatory trigger is acetylcholine.
e. Nitric oxide has an important role in its activity.

1.41 Parasympathetic agonism will lead to the following:

a. Bradycardia.
b. Gut peristalsis.
c. Contraction of urinary bladder sphincter.
d. Uterine contraction.
e. Piloerection.

1.42 Autonomic β_1-adrenergic agonism leads to:

a. Tachycardia.
b. Skeletal muscle vasodilatation.
c. Renin secretion.
d. Lipolysis in fat cells.
e. Cutaneous vasoconstriction.

1.43 Clonidine:

a. Is an α_2-agonist.
b. Is a pro-drug.
c. Has both central and peripheral actions.
d. Reduces the MAC of inhalational anaesthetic agents.
e. Given epidurally counteracts the effect of epidural local anaesthetics.

1.44 The following are non-cardioselective β-adrenergic blocking drugs:

a. Atenolol.
b. Esmolol.
c. Propranolol.
d. Sotalol.
e. Timolol.

1.45 Active post-release re-uptake at their respective neuronal sites is characteristic of the following neurotransmitters:

a. Adrenaline.
b. Acetylcholine.
c. Dopamine.
d. Serotonin.
e. GABA.

1.46 The following are nonapeptides:

a. Vasopressin.
b. Oxytocin.
c. Histamine.
d. Serotonin.
e. Atrial natriuretic peptide.

Pharmacology

1.47   The characteristics of active transmembranal transport include the following:

a. Selectivity.
b. Competitive inhibition by enzymes.
c. Temperature dependence.
d. Saturability.
e. Movement against an electrochemical gradient.

1.48   Glucuronidation as a means of drug metabolism:

a. Is a Phase 1 biotransformation reaction.
b. Occurs in the cytoplasm of hepatocytes.
c. Results in an acidic polar molecule.
d. Renders the drug more lipophilic.
e. Is the primary mode of conjugation of propofol.

1.49   Lipid solubility of drugs is more likely if the drugs have:

a. A hydroxyl (-OH) group.
b. An amide ($-CONH_2$) moiety.
c. A benzene ring.
d. A carboxylic ($-COOH$) group.
e. A halogen radical.

1.50   The side effects of heparin include the following:

a. Thrombocytopenia.
b. Teratogenesis.
c. Osteoporosis.
d. Suppression of aldosterone synthesis in the adrenal cortex.
e. Skin necrosis.

1.51   Protamine sulphate:

a. Is a low-molecular-weight acidic protein.
b. Reverses the effects of heparin by competitive pharmacological antagonism.
c. May have an anticoagulant effect of its own.
d. Can induce a neutropenia.
e. Has been known to produce pulmonary hypertension.

1.52 Anticholinesterases:

a. Are normally oxydiaphoretic inhibitors of acetylcholinesterase.
b. Antagonise acetylcholinesterase by covalent bonding.
c. Are known to block K^+ channels.
d. May increase acetylcholine release from pre-synaptic nerve terminals.
e. Can produce a desensitisation block at the NM junction.

1.53 The following neuromuscular blocking agents produce metabolites that also possess neuromuscular blocking activity:

a. Atracurium.
b. D-tubocurarine.
c. Mivacurium.
d. Pancuronium.
e. Vecuronium.

1.54 The following cause impairment of neuromuscular transmission at skeletal NM junction receptors due to decreased release of acetylcholine at pre-synaptic sites:

a. Aminoglycoside antibiotics.
b. Steroid overdosage.
c. Eaton–Lambert syndrome.
d. Myasthenia gravis.
e. Anticonvulsant administration.

1.55 The following are recognised additives found in IV anaesthetic induction agents:

a. Di-sodium edetate.
b. Sodium carbonate.
c. Benzethonium chloride.
d. Propylene glycol.
e. Tri-acyl glycerides.

1.56 The following IV anaesthetic agents are presented for use as racemic mixtures:

a. Propofol.
b. Thiopentone sodium.
c. Methohexitone.
d. Etomidate.
e. Ketamine.

1.57 Propofol:

a. May contain sodium metabisulphite as an additive.
b. Undergoes significant first-pass metabolism in the lungs.
c. Produces its effects by action at GABA$_B$ receptors.
d. On biotransformation produces a glucuronide as its main metabolite.
e. On biotransformation produces active metabolites.

1.58 Thiopentone sodium:

a. Owes its hypnotic activity to its basic barbiturate ring.
b. Is more lipid soluble than other barbiturates because of the presence of a sulphur atom.
c. Is less than 50% ionised at the pH of blood.
d. Undergoes significant lung uptake in its first circulatory pass.
e. Needs to adopt the enol form tautomer for effective in vivo activity.

1.59 Isoflurane:

a. Is a halogenated alkane.
b. Is a stereo-isomer of enflurane.
c. Is the only halogenated inhalational anaesthetic reputed to cause the 'coronary steal' syndrome.
d. Is regarded as providing brain protection in the event of hypoxia.
e. Is provided for clinical use with a preservative additive.

1.60 The following local anaesthetic agents are presented for clinical use as racemic mixtures:

a. Amethocaine.
b. Lidocaine (lignocaine).
c. Bupivacaine.
d. Prilocaine.
e. Ropivacaine.

1.61 In the case of μ, κ, and δ opioid receptors:

a. They are all G protein-coupled receptors.
b. They are all found in the spinal cord dorsal horn cells.
c. They all mediate analgesic effects.
d. They are all responsible for respiratory depression.
e. They are all involved in the production of dysphoria.

1.62   In the case of fentanyl:

   a. It is a piperidine derivative.
   b. It is structurally related to pethidine.
   c. It is primarily a μ agonist.
   d. It crosses the blood–brain barrier better than morphine.
   e. Its muscle rigidity can be antagonised by naloxone.

1.63   In the case of methadone:

   a. It is primarily a κ opioid agonist.
   b. It is structurally related to dextropropoxyphene.
   c. Its *l*- and *d*-isomers possess equal analgesic potency.
   d. Its *l*-isomer is less addictive than its *d*-isomer.
   e. It can be eliminated more quickly via the kidneys by alkalinisation of the urine.

1.64   Naloxone:

   a. Is a pure opioid antagonist.
   b. Enhances the analgesic effect of morphine.
   c. Is effective on intrathecal administration.
   d. On administration can show the phenomenon of 're-narcotisation'.
   e. May partially antagonise the analgesic effect of ketamine.

1.65   In the case of benzodiazepines:

   a. They exert their actions by activating GABA receptor sites.
   b. They produce their sedative effect by action at the α_2 subunit site of the receptor.
   c. Recovery from their actions usually results from redistribution.
   d. Their anterograde amnesia effect is mediated via action at the α_1 subunit site of the receptor.
   e. In their activity they demonstrate a ceiling effect.

1.66   The following are chiral agents:

   a. Acetylsalicylic acid.
   b. Diclofenac.
   c. Ibuprofen.
   d. Naproxen.
   e. Paracetamol.

1.67 Paracetamol:

    a. Is a pro-drug.
    b. Is more bound to plasma proteins than is aspirin.
    c. Shows cross-hyersensitivity with aspirin.
    d. Can produce renal tubular necrosis.
    e. Is reputed to produce hypoglycaemia.

1.68 **In aspirin overdosage the following acids can accumulate in the body:**

    a. Carbonic acid.
    b. Phosphoric acid.
    c. Sulphuric acid.
    d. Pyruvic acid.
    e. Acetoacetic acid.

1.69 Aspirin:

    a. Is both an ester of acetic acid as well as a derivative of benzoic acid.
    b. Inhibits cyclo-oxygenase as well as lipoxygenase.
    c. Readily crosses both the blood–brain barrier and the placental barrier.
    d. Can lower the body temperature in both normothermic persons and hyperthermic persons.
    e. Is equally effective as an analgesic in both somatic pain and visceral pain.

1.70 Metoclopramide:

    a. Has both central and peripheral actions.
    b. Causes increased secretion of gastric acid.
    c. Increases lower oesophageal sphincter tone.
    d. Is useful in patients with diabetic gastroparesis.
    e. Is reputed to reduce analgesic requirements in patients undergoing prostaglandin-induced termination of pregnancy.

1.71 Concerning adenosine:

    a. It is an endogenous nucleotide.
    b. It is inhibited in its uptake by dipyridamole.
    c. It slows atrioventricular (AV) conduction by increasing K^+ conductance.
    d. It can cause bronchoconstriction in susceptible persons.
    e. Its action is impaired by methylxanthines.

1.72 **Insulin:**

a. Is a disulphide-linked polypeptide.
b. Has a plasma half-life measured in minutes.
c. Is carried in the plasma bound to plasma proteins.
d. Undergoes considerable hepatic first-pass effect.
e. Activates the Na^+–K^+–ATPase pump.

1.73 **The following enhance the secretion of insulin:**

a. α_2-adrenergic stimulation.
b. β_2-adrenergic agonism.
c. Stimulation of α cells of the islets of Langerhans of the pancreas.
d. Vagal stimulation.
e. Vasoactive intestinal peptide (VIP).

1.74 **Oxygen:**

a. Is a nonpolar compound.
b. Has an indefinite half-life in nature.
c. Can be present in the body as a diradical.
d. Interferes with CO_2 estimation by the method of infra-red analysis.
e. Can be made available on the anaesthetic machine in the form of size F cylinders.

1.75 **The following are higher for nitrogen compared with oxygen:**

a. Viscosity.
b. Density.
c. Solubility in plasma.
d. Total volume in the body.
e. Critical temperature.

1.76 **Nitrous oxide:**

a. Can produce loss of consciousness at a concentration of 50%.
b. Can be provided from D cylinders on the anaesthetic machine.
c. Is a recognised triggering agent for malignant hyperpyrexia.
d. Undergoes biotransformation in the body.
e. Can cause elevation of right atrial pressure.

1.77 **The following 'recreational' drugs bring about their effects partly at least by acting at 5HT receptors:**

a. MDMA.
b. Phencyclidine.
c. LSD.
d. Cocaine.
e. Cannabis.

Physics

1.78   In the SI units nomenclature:

   a. The unit of length is defined by reference to the speed of light
      in air.
   b. Mass is the only base quantity that is still defined by reference
      to a physical entity.
   c. The unit of time is defined by reference to the activity of the
      krypton atom.
   d. The candela is the unit of illuminance.
   e. All the units are 'extensive'.

1.79   The following have a relationship in accordance with the 'fourth
       power' law, i.e. they are related to each other thus: $X \propto Y^4$:

   a. *Laminar flow* in a conduit and the *radius* of the conduit.
   b. The *energy* in an oscillating system and the *amplitude* of the
      oscillations.
   c. *Conductance* in an electrical circuit and the *radius* of the
      conducting cable.
   d. The *energy* of electromagnetic radiations and their *kelvin
      temperature*.
   e. The magnitude of the product of *van der Waals' forces* of
      dipole–dipole attractions and their *distance* apart.

1.80   The following are independent of temperature:

   a. Bunsen solubility coefficient.
   b. Osmolality of a solution.
   c. Vapour pressure of a liquid.
   d. Decay of a radioactive isotope.
   e. Latent heat of vaporisation of water.

1.81   The following refer to the same thing:

   a. Ionic chemical bond and electrovalent bond of a chemical
      compound.
   b. Proton number and atomic number of an element.
   c. Natural logarithms and Briggsian logarithms.
   d. Critical temperature and transition temperature.
   e. Dielectric constant and relative permittivity.

1.82   The critical temperature of each of the following gases is below
       0°C:

   a. Oxygen.
   b. Carbon dioxide.
   c. Nitrous oxide.
   d. Nitrogen.
   e. Xenon.

1.83 **The following statements are true:**

a. Oxygen cylinders have a filling ratio that is higher in the tropics than in temperate zones.
b. The pin index system of an anaesthetic machine is foolproof.
c. The Bodok seal on an anaesthetic machine can safely be made of compressed cork.
d. The gauge on a nitrous oxide cylinder gives an accurate idea of the amount of the agent in the cylinder.
e. The contents of a carbon dioxide cylinder are partly in liquid form.

1.84 **The operational voltage in the following is of the order of kilovolts:**

a. AC electricity when generated at a power station.
b. The voltage in a diathermy (electrosurgical) unit.
c. The voltage in an ultrasound scanner unit.
d. The voltage when a CO_2 laser is operational.
e. The voltage of activity of a DC defibrillator.

1.85 **The presence of the following in an electrical wiring system is a guarantee against electrocution from ventricular fibrillation:**

a. A low rated, say 3 A, fuse.
b. An isolated circuit.
c. A line isolation monitor.
d. Rendering the equipment casing at near-zero potential.
e. Presence of a circuit breaker.

1.86 **Bipolar diathermy:**

a. Does not require a 'return electrode'.
b. Is better for 'cutting' mode than is monopolar diathermy.
c. Eliminates the risk of tissue damage from 'channelling'.
d. Is safer in a patient with a cardiac pacemaker than is monopolar diathermy.
e. Is safer for electrocauterizing tissues during laparoscopic procedures.

1.87 **The following are features common to the 'Clark electrode' and the 'fuel cell' as devices for measuring oxygen:**

a. They both require an external source of energy.
b. The metals of their electrodes are the same.
c. The reaction at their cathodes is between the same agents.
d. Temperature is a determinant of the working of both devices.
e. They both have approximately the same response time.

1.88 The chemical reaction involved in each of the following changes is brought about by covalent linkages between the agents concerned:

a. Chelation of Ca^{2+} ions by edetate in blood sample bottles.
b. Conversion of fibrin monomers to firm fibrin by fibrinogen stabilising factor.
c. Neutralisation of heparin by protamine sulphate.
d. Anticholinesterase activity of neostigmine.
e. The inactivation of cyclo-oxygenase by aspirin.

1.89 In the case of the bobbin of an anaesthetics machine rotameter unit:

a. Its proper functioning needs the tube to be rendered antistatic even if no flammable anaesthetic agents are being used.
b. If lost, it is correctly replaceable with another bobbin of the same dimensions.
c. It maintains its position during gas flow solely as the result of the balance of the kinetic energy of upward gas flow and the downward pull on the bobbin of the force of gravity.
d. Its proper performance requires the tube to be inclined slightly from the vertical.
e. The gas flow reading is taken from the bobbin's bottom end.

1.90 In a hyperbaric chamber at 2 atmospheres pressure:

a. An anaesthetic machine will give an actual flow rate higher than that indicated on the flowmeter tube.
b. A 10% oxygen in 90% nitrous oxide will still be 'physiological'.
c. The same concentration setting on a TEC Mark 4 vaporiser will give the same percentage of inhalational agent in the final gas mixture as under normobaric conditions.
d. The orotracheal tube will need less air for a gas tight fit compared with that under normobaric conditions.
e. An undrained pneumothorax is likely to cause more respiratory embarrassment than under normobaric conditions.

1.1 Answers

a. **True**– nerve fibres from olfactory mucous membranes to the olfactory bulbs.
b. **True** – maxillary nerve.
c. **False** – only conveys the middle meningeal vessels.
d. **True** – conveys the vagus nerve and both parts of the accessory nerve, in addition to the jugular vein.
e. **False** – the foramen lacerum conveys the internal carotid artery and its sympathetic plexus and some emissary veins.

1.2 Answers

a. **False**.
b. **True**.
c. **True**.
d. **True**.
e. **False**.

1.3 Answers

a. **False** – there is hardly any superficial fascia in the midline in most persons.
b. **True**.
c. **True**.
d. **False** – the ligamentum denticulatum is a band that passes from the pia mater to the arachnoid mater and dura mater to suspend the spinal cord in the spinal canal.
e. **False** – the pia mater is the innermost of the three meninges and closely invests the spinal cord.

1.4 Answers

a. **False** – they both leave via their respective jugular foramina.
b. **False** – the left recurrent laryngeal nerve arises within the thorax, the right at the level of the subclavian artery.
c. **True** – the rounded superior ganglion is situated on the nerve within the jugular foramen, the cylindrical inferior ganglion lies on the nerve just below the jugular foramen.
d. **False** – mainly the left vagus.
e. **False** – the posterior vagus (which is the 'right' vagus) is the essential contributor of the coeliac branch to the coeliac plexus.

1.5 Answers

a. **False** – the right crus arises from first three lumbar vertebral bodies, the left crus from the first two lumbar vertebral bodies.
b. **False** – its motor supply is solely from the phrenic nerves (C 3, 4 and 5). Its sensory supply to its central part is from the phrenic nerve; the peripheral part is from the lower five intercostal nerves.
c. **False** – More posterior, but anterior to the aortic opening.
d. **False** – the aorta plus thoracic duct and azygos vein.
e. **False** – at the level of the 8th thoracic vertebra, because the vena cava is the anterior-most structure of the trio – vena cava, oesophagus and aorta. Therefore it must penetrate the diaphragm, which is domed, at the higher level, i.e. the 8th thoracic vertebra, compared with the oesophagus, at the 10th vertebral level, and the aorta, at the 12th vertebral level.

1.6 Answers

a. **False** – it is a heterodimer. It consists of an α-subunit, MW c. 100,000, and a β-subunit, MW c. 55,000.
b. **False** – it is an antiport system because the two ions Na^+ and K^+ move in opposite directions.
c. **False** – it is 3–2.
d. **False** – the movement of Na^+ and K^+ through ion channels is much faster because they have to provide for faster activity such as nerve impulse conduction.
e. **True** – cardiac glycosides inhibit the activity of the Na^+–K^+–ATPase pump by preventing the removal of the phosphoryl group from the transport protein, which is an essential step in opening the cell to the outside so as to allow expulsion of Na^+ from the cell. The result is a higher intracellular Na^+ concentration, thus leading to a lowering of the Na^+ gradient from the outside to the inside of the cell. A high Na^+ gradient between the outside and the inside of the cell is necessary to maintain the Na^+–Ca^{2+} antiport pump. In the absence of such a high intracellular Na^+ concentration, Ca^{2+} is retained in the cell in a higher concentration and stimulates cardiac muscle contraction.

1.7 Answers

a. **True** – it depends on the presence of a protein, which mediates as the carrier of the agent across the cell membrane.
b. **False** – it requires no extraneous energy supply.
c. **True** – because the amount of carrier protein is finite.
d. **True** – because the activity of the carrier protein is temperature dependent. Note: all transport processes are temperature dependent, even simple diffusion, because the 'internal energy' of the molecules is a function of temperature.
e. **True**.

1.8 Answers

a. **False** – a simple chemical reaction between the 'acid' carbon dioxide and the 'basic' globin proteins.

b. **False** – CO_2 can be, and is, hydrated in the plasma but by a simple chemical reaction. However, the process is very slow, and the effective conversion of CO_2 to form H_2CO_3 and ultimately $-HCO_3$ takes place inside the red cells, where the presence of carbonic anhydrase accelerates the process a million fold!

c. **False** – atracurium is normally eliminated by Hofmann degradation – spontaneous non-enzymatic breakdown of an agent at physiological temperatures and pH, although it is also eliminable by plasma butyrylcholinesterase activity. Adolf Wilhelm Hofmann (1818–1892) described the process in 1851.

d. **True** – produced by nitric oxide synthase acting on arginine, converting it to citrulline in the process.

e. **True** – requires pyruvate kinase.

1.9 Answers

a. **True** – it has four pyrrole groups in each haem moiety.

b. **True** – allosterism is a property of enzymes or proteins whereby the binding of substrate to one active site can affect the properties of other active sites in the same enzyme or protein molecule. Where such binding facilitates further enzymic activity the phenomenon is called *positive* cooperativity, where it inhibits further binding, *negative* cooperativity. In the case of oxygen and haemoglobin it is one of positive cooperativity; this helps to make its binding with O_2 a 'positive feedback' mechanism.

c. **True** – 27 mmHg (c. 3.5 kPa) compared with 20 mmHg (c. 2.67 kPa) for HbF. The P_{50} is that partial pressure of O_2 at which haemoglobin is 50% saturated with oxygen.

d. **True**.

e. **True**.

1.10 Answers

a. **True** – the ratio of the combining power of O_2 (in millilitres) with haemoglobin (in grams). It is normally 1.34 ml/g.

b. **True** – shift to the left of the haemoglobin oxygen dissociation curve in stored blood, resulting from a diminution in 2,3 DPG.

c. **False** – reduction in alveolar concentration of a gas and therefore reduced uptake because of dilution effect of another gas. Common cause of 'diffusion' hypoxia at the end of an anaesthetic when nitrous oxide leaves the tissues for the alveolar space. Named after Bernard Raymond Fink of Seattle, who first described it in the 1920s.

d. **False** – Fahraeus–Lindqvist effect – reduction in viscosity of blood as it flows in smaller bore vessels because of the tendency of the red cells to align themselves in a regular manner in the vessel lumen. As such it is a property of the cells themselves and not of the haemoglobin within them.

e. **True** – Rapaport–Luebering shunt – the shunt in the Embden–Meyerhof (glycolytic) pathway that leads to the formation of 2,3 DPG (diphosphoglycerate). The percentage of haemoglobin molecules containing 2,3 DPG governs the overall P_{50} of haemoglobin.

1.11 Answers

a. **True** – the combination of oxygen with haemoglobin facilitates the further combination of oxygen. This is akin to the combination of substrate molecules with the active site of an enzyme, leading to the binding of small signal molecules at sites distinct from the active site yet triggering conformational changes that are transmitted to the active site. This is an example of *positive cooperativity* (see **9b**.)

b. **False** – it is one of oxygenation. Oxidation is a process of addition of protons or removal of electrons. In oxidation the substrate (in this case the iron moiety of haem) loses electrons and the iron takes the ferric (Fe^{3+}) form, converting the haemoglobin to methaemoglobin. In oxygenation it gains (a molecule of) oxygen.

c. **False** – occurs at the 6th coordination position. In haemoglobin the Fe^{2+} has six coordination positions, four of which are attached to the nitrogen atom of each of the four pyrrole moieties. The 5th is attached to an imidazole ring of a histidine residue and in reduced haemoglobin the 6th position remains unoccupied. In oxyhaemoglobin it is this 6th position that is combined with oxygen.

d. **True**.

e. **False** – oxygenation of haemoglobin makes the Fe^{2+} ion less magnetic, a property which is utilised in magnetic resonance imaging of the brain to study brain activity.

1.12 Answers

a. **True** – carbonic anhydrase is found in seven forms in the body. The carbonic anhydrase II form is present in high concentration in red cells.

b. **True** – zinc is an essential metal in many enzymes, including alcohol dehydrogenase.

c. **True** – as the pH falls its activity is reduced.

d. **False** – although the zinc atom in carbonic anhydrase has three coordination sites occupied by the imidazole rings of three histidine residues, it is the fourth coordination site bound to a water molecule that is responsible for the activity of the enzyme.

e. **True** – c. 10^6 to 10^7 times faster.

1.13 Answers

a. **True** – they are most lax in the duodenum and tightest in the colon.

b. **True**.

c. **True**.

d. **False** – the jejunum normally absorbs about 4 L/day, the ileum about 2 L.

e. **True**.

1.14 Answers

a. **True** – c. 285–290 mosmol/L.

b. **True** – c. 135–138 mosmol/L.

c. **False** – CSF has about 40% less K^+ – CSF: 2.9 mmol/L; plasma: 4.5 mmol/L.

d. **False** – CSF has about 15% more chloride than plasma.

e. **False** – CSF has about 30% less glucose – CSF: c. 3.5 mmol/L; plasma: c. 4.0–4.5 mmol/L.

1.15 Answers

a. **False** – diaphragmatic contraction has the predominant role. The intercostals also play a part.

b. **True**.

c. **True** – usually about 2–3%.

d. **True** – to overcome the elastic recoil of the lungs and chest wall.

e. **False** – a passive process resulting from elastic recoil of the lungs and chest wall and utilising the potential energy stored in them during the inspiratory phase.

1.16 Answers

a. **False** – it becomes less negative.
b. **True**.
c. **True**.
d. **False** – because the blood flow increase is greater compared with the increase in ventilation.
e. **True** – the mean capillary pressure is as follows: at the top: c. 0.8 kPa; in the middle of the lung: c. 2.2 kPa; at the bottom: c. 3.5 kPa.

1.17 Answers

a. **False** – about 90% dipalmitoyl phosphatidyl choline (dipalmitoyl lecithin). The rest are proteins and carbohydrates.
b. **False** – Type II cells, containing lamellated osmophilic bodies c. 0.5–1.0 μm in diameter.
c. **False** – about 15–30 hours.
d. **True** – antioxidants slow the rate of oxidation reactions, some by acting as chelating agents to sequester metal ions that catalyse oxidation reactions, others by inhibiting the oxidation reaction by removing oxygen free radicals. Biological antioxidants include vitamin E and β-carotene.
e. **True** – by reducing the intra-alveolar negative pressure and thereby preventing transudation of fluid into the alveoli.

1.18 Answers

a. **False** – the volume of air exhaled in 1 second starting from a full inspiration.
b. **True**.
c. **False** – It should exceed 75% in the normal subject.
d. **True**.
e. **False** – because airway obstruction by increasing the airway resistance makes the forcing out of air more difficult and therefore requires more time.

1.19 Answers

a. **True**.
b. **False** – occurs mainly in pulmonary arterioles of c. 200 μm internal diameter. These vessels are more advantageously positioned in close relation to smaller bronchioles and alveoli and are therefore capable of more rapid and accurate detection of hypoxia.
c. **False** – it is a localised response, see **b**.
d. **True**.
e. **False** – is aggravated by hypercapnia.

1.20 Answers

a. **True**.
b. **True** – the blood flow in each (2 mg) carotid body is c. 0.04 ml/minute, i.e. c. 2000 ml per 100 g/minute tissue. Brain: 0.55 ml; heart c. 80 ml; liver c. 100 ml; kidneys: c. 400 ml.
c. **True**.
d. **True**.
e. **False** – Type I cells, which are glomus cells. They are round cells roughly 10 μm in diameter and present in clusters.

1.21 Answers

a. **False** – from thoracic segments 1–4.
b. **False** – under parasympathetic (vagal) domination.
c. **True** – there is little, if any, parasympathetic supply to the ventricles.
d. **False** – from the left vagus nerve. The right vagus supplies the sinoatrial node.
e. **False** – there are α adrenergic components as well.

1.22 Answers

a. **False**.
b. **False**.
c. **True**.
d. **True**.
e. **True**.

Note – 'fast' action potentials are the result of the opening of fast sodium channels, which occurs in phase 0 of the action potential, and are responsible for the rapid spike-like onset of the action potential. In the case of the SA node and AV node action potentials the 'resting' potential is less negative, only –55 mV. At this level of negativity, the fast sodium channels have essentially become 'inactivated' and only the slow calcium-sodium channels can open. Hence the slower action potential.

1.23 Answers

a. **True** – –55 to –60 mV, compared with –85 to –90 mV for the ventricular muscle cell.
b. **False** – has a less steep upstroke.
c. **True**.
d. **False** – the depolarisation is more gradual.
e. **True** – because tetrodotoxin blocks sodium channels, but the upstroke of the SA node action potential is not produced by fast sodium channels. The latter have essentially become 'inactivated' at the level of negativity –55 to –60 mV of the 'resting' potential of the SA node.

1.24 Answers

a. True – increase in venous return leads to increased activation of atrial stretch receptors leading to a tachycardia and increased cardiac output. It does not occur in the transplanted heart because of denervation.

b. True – stimulation of ventricular stretch receptors leads to hypotension and bradycardia.

c. False – laryngospasm resulting from stimulation of a 'remote' site such as the anus or the uterine cervix.

d. True – rise in intracranial pressure leads to diminution of cerebral perfusion and hypoxia of the vasomotor centre. This leads to hypertension with a compensatory bradycardia.

e. False – lung inflation leads to activation of pulmonary stretch receptors, which via the vagus inhibits activity of respiratory muscles and brings inspiration to a halt.

1.25 Answers

a. True – its normal O_2 utilisation is 8.7 ml per 100 g/minute. The values for other organs are as follows: brain: 3.5; kidneys: 6.7; liver: 3.5; skeletal muscle: 0.15. With strenuous exercise the skeletal muscle O_2 utilisation is c. 12 ml per 100 g, the heart's is 15–20 ml.

b. True – Brain (jugular venous bulb): c. 65%; heart coronary sinus: c. 40%.

c. True – the total blood volume that the heart can accommodate (at the end of diastole) is about 550 ml. If the stroke volume is about 70 ml and is about 60–70% of the ventricular end-diastolic volume, then the latter is about 100–120 ml. Therefore the total blood volume of the two ventricles is about 240 ml. Therefore the atria must hold about 270–300 ml.

d. False – under basal conditions only c. 35% of the calorie needs of the heart is met by glucose; 60% is met by fat and the rest by ketones and amino acids.

e. True – normally less than 1% of the energy is dependent on anaerobic metabolism, but it can rise to c.10% under hypoxic conditions.

1.26 Answers

a. True.

b. True.

c. True.

d. False – a falsely lower reading.

e. True.

1.27 Answers

a. **False** – it is higher in the femoral and dorsalis pedis arteries than in the aorta.
b. **False** – diastolic pressure decreases with increasing distance from the heart.
c. **True** – because the decrease in diastolic pressure is greater than the increase in systolic pressure.
d. **False** – the pulse wave peaks as it moves down the arterial tree.
e. **False** – it is much higher because of separation from the ventricles by the aortic valves.

1.28 Answers

a. **True**.
b. **True**.
c. **True**.
d. **True**.
e. **True**.

1.29 Answers

a. **True** – because the Na^+–K^+–ATPase pump has been rendered dysfunctional.
b. **True**.
c. **False** – a rise in cerebral perfusion pressure will help maintain blood flow and to that extent reduce the degree of ischaemic damage.
d. **True**.
e. **True**.

1.30 Answers

a. **True** – thiopentone reduces the portion of metabolic activity responsible for neuronal signalling and impulse traffic, but not the portion responsible for basal metabolic function, i.e. the component responsible for cellular integrity, the 'housekeeping' component.
b. **True**.
c. **True**.
d. **True**.
e. **False**.

1.31 Answers

a. **False** – hepatic artery: c. 20–25%: 300 ml/minute; portal vein: c. 75–80%: 1200 ml/minute.
b. **True** – c. 25 ml from each supply.
c. **False** – arteries: 20%; capillaries: 10%; veins: 70%.
d. **False** – only for 24–48 hours.
e. **False** – c. 20% of adult haem production is in the liver.

1.32 Answers

a. **True** – edetate chelates calcium and thereby maintains the blood in its fluid state.
b. **True** – chelates copper (Wilson's disease), mercury, zinc and lead (in heavy metal poisoning) and promotes their excretion in urine.
c. **False** – protamine sulphate is a strongly basic polycationic protein that by ionically binding to the acidic polyanionic heparin forms a stable salt devoid of any anticoagulant activity.
d. **True** – desferrioxamine chelates iron (but not calcium) in thalassaemic patients during blood transfusion.
e. **False** – edrophonium acts by combining with acetylcholinesterase by electrostatic bonding.

Note: the word 'chelation' comes from the Greek *chela*, meaning 'claw', and indicates the manner in which metals ions are rendered 'impotent' by being bound to the 'lone pair' electrons of the chelating agent. The agent 'claws' itself onto the metal ion and incorporates it into a moiety in its structure, thereby removing the metal's ionised status and thus its activity.

1.33 Answers

a. **False** – the 'brownness' is caused by an iron containing cytochrome that only becomes apparent after fat depletion.
b. **False** – found in the fetus from about 22 weeks' gestation.
c. **True** – in relation to large veins so that the heat generated can be carried away to other parts of the body.
d. **True**.
e. **True**. In normal fat cells ATP generation in mitochondria depends on the inner mitochondrial membrane being impermeable to protons, thus compelling the latter to enter the mitochondrial matrix only via the ATP-generating channels and thus produce chemical energy. In the case of brown fat cells a special protein, thermogenin, acts as a channel – 'a hole in the wall' – allowing the proton to flow through and thereby short-circuit the ATP-generating process. Thus with thermogenin no ATP need be produced, only heat.

1.34 Answers

a. **True**.
b. **True**.
c. **True**.
d. **True**.
e. **True**.

1.35 Answers

a. False – only a very small amount of CO_2 is carried in the blood as carbonic acid.
b. False – by combining with the amino acids of the globin chains.
c. True – by combining with the amino acids of plasma proteins.
d. True – by the histidine moieties of the globin chains.
e. True – c. 70% of the blood CO_2 is in the form of bicarbonate.

1.36 Answers

a. True.
b. False – water specific density: 1.0; alcohol: 0.8.
c. False – although alcohol is readily absorbed from the stomach, absorption is higher in the small intestine because of the greater surface area.
d. True.
e. True.

1.37 Answers

a. False – their pHs are as follows: H-S: c. 6.0; N-S: c. 5. 5%;G: c. 4; G-S: c. 4.5.
b. False – see **a** above.
c. False – has lactate as buffer.
d. False – G-S also has 'free water'. Free water is the water content of a solution that is not matched by equivalent ions to make it near-iso-osmolar with plasma. Note: strictly speaking, none of the solutions is iso-osmolar with plasma because their osmolarities are about 278–285 compared with that of plasma, which is about 285–290 mosmol/L. Therefore all of them have some 'free water'. (See **e** below).
e. True – their osmolarities are c. 5 mosmol less than that of plasma (see **d**.)

1.38 Answers

a. True.
b. False.
c. False.
d. True.
e. False.

The two essential attributes required of an insufflating gas are: (i) it must be highly soluble in blood; and (ii) it must be inert or at least 'physiological'. CO_2 meets both these requirements. N_2O can be used, and has been used in the past, provided: (i) it is not used simultaneously as an anaesthetic agent; and (ii) no diathermy or laser is used. N_2O explodes at about 400°C. Helium too has been used, but it is insoluble and therefore can cause 'gas embolism'.

1.39 Answers

a. **False** – the definition of a 'muscarinic effect' is 'that effect that is blocked by atropine'. Atropine does not act at ganglionic sites.
b. **False** – also includes those effects at all autonomic ganglia.
c. **True** – see **a** above.
d. **False** – phenoxybenzamine is an α-adrenergic blocker.
e. **False** – it is the other way round. Nicotinic effects are always linked to changes in ion permeability, while muscarinic effects are not necessarily so linked. An ion permeability-linked effect is generally faster than one not linked to ion permeability.

1.40 Answers

a. **True**.
b. **True**.
c. **False**.
d. **True**.
e. **True**.

1.41 Answers

a. **True** – vagal effect.
b. **True**.
c. **False** – normally mediated by α_{1A} agonism.
d. **False** – normally mediated by α_1 agonism.
e. **False** – it is a sympathetic effect, although cholinergic in nature.

1.42 Answers

a. **True**.
b. **False** – β_2-adrenergic effect.
c. **True**.
d. **True**.
e. **False** – α_1 effect.

1.43 Answers

a. **True**.
b. **False**.
c. **True** – centrally, clonidine is a potent α_2 agonist at medullary receptors, resulting in diminished sympathetic outflow and therefore a fall in blood pressure. It also directly stimulates α_2 receptors in peripheral arterioles, causing further hypotension.
d. **True**.
e. **False** – it potentiates epidural local anaesthetics.

1.44 Answers

a. **False**.
b. **False**.
c. **True**.
d. **True**.
e. **True**.

1.45 Answers

a. **True**.
b. **False** – acetylcholine is immediately broken down by acetylcholinesterase into choline and acetate. The choline undergoes re-uptake, not acetylcholine.
c. **True**.
d. **True**.
e. **True**.

1.46 Answers

a. **True**.
b. **True** – differs from vasopressin with respect to just two amino acids; this is why each of the two shows about 20% of the pharmacological activity of the other.
c. **False** – histamine is a substituted imidazole.
d. **False** – serotonin is 5-hydroxytryptamine, a substituted mono amino acid.
e. **False** – atrial natriuretic peptide is a 28-amino acid peptide.

1.47 Answers

a. **True**.
b. **True**.
c. **True**.
d. **True**.
e. **True**.

1.48 Answers

a. **False** – it is the chief method of Phase 2 biotransformation reactions.
b. **False** – although most Phase 2 transformations occur in the cytoplasm, glucuronidation occurs in the endoplasmic reticulum.
c. **True**.
d. **False** – more hydrophilic.
e. **True** – both propofol itself as well as its hydroxylate –2,6 di-isopropyl 1,4 quinol – undergo glucuronidation.

1.49   **Answers**

    a. **False**.
    b. **False**.
    c. **True**.
    d. **False**.
    e. **True**.

1.50   **Answers**

    a. **True**.
    b. **False**.
    c. **True**.
    d. **True**.
    e. **False** – side effect of warfarin.

1.51   **Answers**

    a. **False** – LMW basic protein.
    b. **False** – by chemical antagonism – neutralisation by ionic binding of its basic site to the acidic polyionic site of heparin to form a stable salt that has no anticoagulant effect of its own.
    c. **True** – protamine has two active sites, one that binds to heparin and the other that exerts a mild anticoagulant effect of its own.
    d. **True** – but it is transient.
    e. **True** – causes pulmonary vasoconstriction and right ventricular strain.

1.52   **Answers**

    a. **True** – all except edrophonium.
    b. **True**.
    c. **True**.
    d. **True**.
    e. **True** – by producing high concentrations of acetylcholine at the receptor site.

1.53 Answers

a. **False** – atracurium is broken down into laudanosine and a related quaternary acid, neither of which has neuromuscular blocking properties.

b. **False** – d-tubocurarine is not metabolised. 50–60% of the injected agent is excreted in the urine. The rest is probably excreted in the bile.

c. **False** – mivacurium is hydrolysed by butyrylcholinesterase to a quaternary monoester, which is then broken down into a dicarboxylic acid. Neither has neuromuscular blocking activity.

d. **True** – the 3-OH metabolite of pancuronium has about two-thirds the potency of the parent agent.

e. **True** – the 3-OH metabolite has about 80% the potency of the parent compound and is regarded as the reason for delayed recovery after long-term use of vecuronium in ITU patients.

1.54 Answers

a. **True** – aminoglycoside antibiotics also depress postjunctional sensitivity to acetylcholine.

b. **False** – steroids increase acetylcholine release at pre-synaptic motor terminals.

c. **True** – as a result of an autoimmune disorder caused by antibodies directed against Ca^{2+} channels.

d. **False** – in myasthenia gravis the defect results from antibodies targeted against the α-subunit of the postsynaptic membrane.

e. **True** – by depressing the release of acetylcholine. But anticonvulsants may actually increase the need for higher doses of neuromuscular blocking agents (NMBAs) because of increased binding to plasma proteins.

1.55 Answers

a. **True** – present in propofol (0.005%) as a bacteriostatic.

b. **True** – 6% $Na_2 CO_3$ is present in thiopentone sodium to prevent formation of free acid on exposure of the agent to air.

c. **True** – in ketamine.

d. **True** – in etomidate as a solubilising agent.

e. **True** – in propofol as medium- and long-chain triglycerides as emulsifying agents.

1.56 Answers

a. **False** – propofol is an achiral agent.

b. **True**.

c. **True**.

d. **True**.

e. **True**.

1.57 Answers

a. **True** – in preparations in the USA.
b. **True** – about 30%.
c. **False** – acts at $GABA_A$ receptors.
d. **True**.
e. **False**.

1.58 Answers

a. **False** – its hypnotic activity is due to its alkyl side chains.
b. **False** – the sulphur atom gives the agent a more rapid onset and shorter duration of action.
c. **True** – c. 40%.
d. **True** – c. 17%.
e. **True** – through keto-enol tautomerism the S atom assumes the enol form. This allows for the water-soluble form of the agent in its alkaline form, thus permitting its IV use.

1.59 Answers

a. **False** – it is a halogenated ether. Halothane is the only halogenated alkane.
b. **False** – it is a structural isomer of enflurane.
c. **True** – although enflurane has been similarly implicated the accepted view is that enflurane does not produce the syndrome.
d. **True**.
e. **False** – halothane is the only one that contains a preservative viz. 0.01% thymol.

1.60 Answers

a. **False** – amethocaine is an achiral agent.
b. **False** – Lidocaine is an achiral agent.
c. **True** – it is also available as an S-enantiomer, levobupivacaine.
d. **True**.
e. **False** – ropivacaine is a chiral compound, but is provided for use as a pure S-enantiomer.

1.61 Answers

a. **True**.
b. **True**.
c. **True**.
d. **False** – respiratory depression is mediated through μ and δ opioid receptors.
e. **False** – dysphoria is mediated through κ receptors.

1.62 Answers

a. **True**.
b. **True**.
c. **True**.
d. **True**.
e. **True**.

1.63 Answers

a. **False** – it is primarily a μ opioid agonist.
b. **True**.
c. **False** – the analgesic activity of the racemate of methadone is almost entirely attributable to *l*-methadone, which is almost 50 times as potent as the *d* form.
d. **False** – it is the *d*-isomer that is less addictive.
e. **False** – it is more easily eliminable by acidification of the urine.

1.64 Answers

a. **True**.
b. **True**.
c. **True**.
d. **True** – because its effect is shorter lived than that of morphine.
e. **True**.

1.65 Answers

a. **False** – they act by blocking the action by the natural ligand at the receptor site.
b. **False** – sedative effect is due to activity at the α_1 subunit. Anxiolysis is due to activity at the α_2 subunit.
c. **True**.
d. **True**.
e. **True** – because of **a**.

1.66 Answers

a. **False**.
b. **False**.
c. **True** – ibuprofen is presented as a mixture of two enantiomers, R (−) and S (+), of which the S (+) is the main anti-inflammatory form.
d. **True**.
e. **False**.

1.67 Answers

a. **False** – but it is an active metabolite of the now obsolete drug phenacetin.
b. **False** – aspirin is c. 80–90% bound to plasma proteins, paracetamol only c. 20–50% bound.
c. **False** – paracetamol can be given safely to patients allergic to aspirin.
d. **True** – especially in overdosage.
e. **True** – which can lead to coma.

1.68 Answers

a. **True** – due to increased O_2 consumption and CO_2 production.
b. **True** – impaired renal function leads to accumulation of phosphoric acids.
c. **True** – impaired renal function leads to accumulation of sulphuric acid.
d. **True** – due to derangement of carbohydrate metabolism.
e. **True** – due to derangement of carbohydrate metabolism.

1.69 Answers

a. **True** – it is the salicylic ester of acetic acid as well as an acetyl derivative of benzoic acid.
b. **False** – it inhibits cyclo-oxygenase but not lipoxygenase.
c. **True**.
d. **False** – it does not have an antipyretic effect in normothermic persons.
e. **False** – aspirin is effective in 'integumental' somatic pain but is ineffective in visceral pain.

1.70 Answers

a. **True** – central action: anti-dopaminergic; peripheral action: muscarinic.
b. **False**.
c. **True** – by a muscarinic effect (see **a.**)
d. **True** – because it increases gastric tone and thereby enhances gastric emptying.
e. **True**.

1.71 Answers

a. **False** – it is an endogenous nucleoside, because it is a combination of adenine, a nucleotide, and ribose, a pentose sugar.
b. **True** – this leads to potentiation of its effects.
c. **True** – by activating acetylcholine-sensitive K^+ channels.
d. **True**.
e. **True** – because methylxanthines block adenosine receptors.

1.72 Answers

a. **True** – insulin is a 5800 Da polypeptide consisting of two amino acid chains with a total of 51 amino acids linked by two intersubunit and one intrasubunit disulphide bonds.
b. **True** – c. 5–6 minutes.
c. **False** – is carried in the plasma as the free monomer.
d. **True** – c. 50% of insulin in the portal vein is inactivated in the liver by insulinase, to a lesser extent in the kidneys and muscle, and slightly in most other tissues.
e. **True**.

1.73 Answers

a. **False** – inhibits.
b. **True**.
c. **False** – the cells of the islet of Langerhans are: α cells (25% of the cells), which secrete glucagon; β cells: c. 60% secrete insulin; d cells: c. 10% secrete somatostatin; and PP cells present in small numbers, which secrete pancreatic polypeptide.
d. **True**.
e. **True** – VIP is a polypeptide secreted by the intestinal mucosa which as its name suggests is a vasodilator and also inhibits gastric secretion.

1.74 Answers

a. **True**.
b. **True** – if not, the human and animal species will not be able to exist in perpetuity.
c. **True** – a diradical is an atom which contains two unpaired electrons.
d. **True** – although oxygen cannot be estimated by infra-red analysis, it nevertheless interferes with CO_2 estimation by that method.
e. **False** – oxygen cylinders of size F (and larger) have no pin index attachments and are too tall for attachment to an anaesthetic machine.

1.75 Answers

a. **False** – viscosity of O_2 (at 25°C) – 0.0208 mPa s; for N_2: 0.0179.
b. **False** – density of O_2 (at 1 bar and 15°C) – 1.337 kg m^{-3}; of N_2: 1.169 kg m^{-3}.
c. **False** – Oswald solubility coefficient of O_2 (at 25°): 0.0310; for N_2: 0.0160.
d. **True** – the total volume of O_2 in the body is not much more than 1 L. The lungs alone contain more than 1 L of N_2.
e. **False** – the critical temperature of N_2 is 123 K; of O_2 it is 155 K.

1.76 Answers

a. **True** – although most patients lose consciousness at a N_2O concentration of c. 80%, some lose consciousness even at 30%.

b. **True** – the usual cylinder size is E, but C and D cylinders too can be attached to an anaesthetic machine because they all have pin index outlets.

c. **False** – unlike the halogenated inhalational anaesthetic agents, N_2O is not reputed to trigger malignant hyperpyrexia.

d. **False** – undergoes no known biotransformation.

e. **True** – N_2O causes pulmonary vasoconstriction and the resulting pulmonary hypertension can cause a rise in right atrial pressure.

1.77 Answers

a. **True** – usually in higher dosage.

b. **False** – it acts at NMDA-type receptors.

c. **True** – mainly a $5HT_2$ receptor agonist on autoreceptors of neurons of raphe nuclei.

d. **True** – cocaine blocks serotonin re-uptake at 5HT receptors, in addition to its effects at dopaminergic and noradrenaline receptors.

e. **False** – acts at a 'cannabinoid' receptor, for which the endogenous ligand is anandamide, an arachidonic acid derivative.

1.78 Answers

a. **False** – by reference to the speed of light in a vacuum.

b. **True** – by reference to a cylinder of platinum–iridium in the International Bureau of Weights and Measures in Sevres, near Paris. However, there are moves to redefine the kilogram by reference to the mass of a number of atoms of an element (e.g. silicon).

c. **False** – by reference to ^{133}caesium, i.e. the time taken for the oscillator, which will force the caesium atom to perform a specified transition, to complete 9,192,631,770 oscillations.

d. **False** – candela is the unit of 'intensity of illumination'. 'Illuminance' (and 'luminance') are different physical 'quantities'.

e. **False** – temperature is not an 'extensive' quantity, i.e. unlike the other quantities, it does not possess 'positive fiduciary marks'; it is not additive. If two fluids at different temperatures are mixed, their combined temperature is not the sum of their original individual temperatures.

An 'extensive' property is one whose magnitude depends on the amount of the substance present in a given thermodynamic state.

I.79 Answers

a. **True** – this is in accordance with the Hagen–Poiseuille equation.
b. **False** – the energy is proportional to the square of the amplitude.
c. **False** – conductance is proportional to the cross-sectional area of the conductor and therefore proportional to the *square* of the radius.
d. **True** – energy is proportional to K^4 in accordance with the Stefan–Boltzmann equation:

$E = s \times K^4$

where s is the Stefan constant.

e. **False** – the force is *inversely* proportional to the 7th power of the distance apart.

I.80 Answers

a. **False** – the solubility of a gas in a liquid decreases with a rise in its temperature.
b. **True** – because osmolality is defined by reference to the number of osmoles per *kilogram* of solvent (water), and 'mass' is independent of temperature. cx. Osmolarity, which is the number of osmoles of solute per *litre* of solution. 'Volume' is temperature dependent.
c. **False** – the higher the temperature the higher the vapour pressure.
d. **True**.
e. **False** – the lower the temperature at which water evaporates, the higher the latent heat of vaporisation.

I.81 Answers

a. **True** – a bond that arises between two atoms when there is a donation of an electron by one atom to the other. The first acquires a positive charge (cation) and the other a negative charge (anion), both assuming the electron configuration of a noble gas. Where electrons are shared the bond is a 'covalent' bond.
b. **True** – the atomic number of an element is determined by the number of protons in its nucleus.
c. **False** – natural logarithms are Napierian logarithms, after John Napier of Edinburgh. Briggsian logarithms, named after William Briggs of Oxford, are logarithms to the base 10.
d. **False** – 'critical' temperature – the temperature above which a gas cannot be liquefied by pressure alone. 'Transition' temperature is: (i) the temperature at which one crystalline form changes to another; (ii) the temperature below which a material becomes a superconductor, (iii) the temperature at which a metal loses its ferromagnetic property and becomes merely paramagnetic (also known as the Curie temperature, after Pierre Curie).
e. **True** – they both are a measure of the ease with which current will flow in the 'dielectric', i.e. the medium between the two plates of a capacitor, which medium may be air or even a vacuum.

1.82 **Answers**

    a. **True** – –118°C.
    b. **False** – 31.04°C.
    c. **False** –36.4°C.
    d. **True** – –146°C.
    e. **False** – 16.5°C.

1.83 **Answers**

    a. **False** – filling ratios are applicable only to cylinders whose contents are a mixture of gas and liquid. The contents of oxygen cylinders are wholly gaseous at room temperature.
    b. **False** – the system can be rendered invalid by: (i) sawing off the pins; (ii) using multiple washers (Bodok seals), or (iii) by connecting the cylinders upside down.
    c. **False** – Bodok seals must be made of nonflammable material.
    d. **False** – because the contents are partly in liquid form, the amount of the agent in the cylinder can be determined only by weighing the cylinder.
    e. **True** – because the agent's critical temperature (31.04°C) is above room temperature.

1.84 **Answers**

    a. **True** – the generated voltage is about 25,000 V. The initial transmission voltage is about 250,000–400,000.
    b. **True** – about 5000–10,000.
    c. **False** – it is the usual mains 240 voltage.
    d. **False** – it is the usual mains 240 voltage.
    e. **True** – it is about 3000–5000.

1.85 **Answers**

There is no absolute guarantee against the deleterious effects of electricity.

    a. **False** – a 3 ampere fuse will protect the appliance against damage by fire, but will not protect a person handling the appliance against VF.
    b. **False**.
    c. **False**.
    d. **False** – microshock delivered directly to the heart as through a pacemaker cable can cause VF.
    e. **False** – a lot depends on the nature of the circuit breaker.

1.86 Answers

a. **False** – both forms of diathermy require a return pathway. In the case of monopolar, it runs from the diathermy plate to the electrosurgical unit. In the case of bipolar the return path runs directly from the surgical forceps to the electrosurgical unit.

b. **False** – cutting is best with monopolar diathermy.

c. **True** – 'channelling' is the phenomenon whereby the diathermy current returns to the machine along an attenuated pathway and in the process causes thermal damage to it.

d. **True** – because the current does not need to traverse the patient's body.

e. **True** – because it will eliminate the likelihood of 'channelling'.

1.87 Answers

a. **False** – the Clark electrode needs one, the fuel cell generates its own energy.

b. **False** – Clark electrode: Ag/AgCl and platinum. Fuel cell: lead anode, gold cathode.

c. **True** – O_2 combines with water as follows:

$$O_2 + 4e + 2\,H_2O = 4(OH)^-$$

d. **True**.

e. **False** – the fuel cell oxygen sensor has a slower response time.

1.88 Answers

a. **True** – it is a 'dative covalent bond'.

b. **True**.

c. **False** – see the MCQ 51 on 'protamine sulphate'.

d. **True** – neostigmine inactivates acetylcholinesterase by carbamylation of the enzyme by covalently bonding with it.

e. **True** – the acetyl moiety of aspirin (acetyl salicylic acid) combines with a serine residue of cyclo-oxygenase by covalent bonding.

1.89 Answers

a. **True**: so as to prevent the bobbin sticking to the tube during rotation.

b. **False**: the new bobbin must be exactly matched with regard to dimensions, mass and surface consistency.

c. **False**: there is also a small upward force, resulting from a slight 'negative' pressure just above the bobbin.

d. **False**.

e. **False**: from the top end.

1.90 Answers

a. **True**.

b. **True** – because the pO_2 will be 10% of 200 kPa 2 atmospheres, which is equal to 20% at 100 kPa, which is the same as in normobaric atmospheric air.

c. **True** – because the saturated vapour pressure of the agent will be the same.

d. **False** – it will need more air to distend it against a 'background' pressure of 2 atmospheres.

e. **True** – because its gases will be at a pressure of 2 bar.

Practice paper 2

Anatomy

2.1 The following statements are true with respect to the heart:

    a. The heart is situated opposite the middle four thoracic vertebrae.
    b. The sympathetic supply is normally from T1 to T4 segments.
    c. The right border on radiological view is formed predominantly by the right ventricular border.
    d. The left coronary artery provides the main supply to the posterior aspect of the left ventricle.
    e. The atrioventricular node is normally innervated by the right vagus nerve.

2.2 The following nerves are entirely sensory in function:

    a. Lateral femoral cutaneous nerve of the thigh.
    b. Ilio-inguinal nerve.
    c. Genitofemoral nerve.
    d. Infra-orbital branch of the mandibular nerve.
    e. Supratrochlear nerve.

2.3 The following nerves provide a cutaneous supply to the head:

    a. Facial nerve.
    b. Maxillary nerve.
    c. First cervical nerve.
    d. Spinal part of the accessory nerve.
    e. Vagus nerve.

2.4 Features of stellate ganglion block include:

    a. Ipsilateral exophthalmos.
    b. Contralateral hypohidrosis.
    c. Ipsilateral complete ptosis.
    d. Contralateral relative mydriasis.
    e. Ipsilateral nasal congestion.

2.5   The following structures run in the lumen of the cavernous sinus:

a. Internal carotid artery.
b. Abducens nerve.
c. Oculomotor nerve.
d. Trochlear nerve.
e. Maxillary nerve.

2.6   The blood–brain barrier is highly permeable to:

a. Water.
b. Sodium.
c. Oxygen.
d. Carbon dioxide.
e. Alcohol.

2.7   The formation of carbaminohaemoglobin:

a. Is per se an enzyme-dependent process.
b. Depends on the presence of 'terminal' amino groups in the haemoglobin molecule.
c. Is markedly pH dependent.
d. Is enhanced by the presence of 2,3 di-phosphoglycerate.
e. Necessitates prior hydration of CO_2 to H_2CO_3.

2.8   The following are phenomena associated with activity inside red cells:

a. Bert effect.
b. Bernoulli phenomenon.
c. Bohr effect.
d. Hamburger phenomenon.
e. Fink effect.

2.9   Ethanol:

a. Acts predominantly by augmenting GABA-mediated synaptic inhibition.
b. Produces vasodilatation solely by a direct action on blood vessels.
c. Decreases the concentration of high-density lipoproteins in the plasma.
d. Activates voltage-gated L-type Ca^{2+} channels.
e. Inhibits adenosine transport.

2.10   Other things being equal, the effects of alcohol come on more quickly:

    a. If taken on an empty stomach.
    b. If taken aerated with carbon dioxide.
    c. If taken with aspirin.
    d. If taken along with metoclopramide.
    e. In women compared with men.

2.11   The following are higher in the cerebrospinal fluid compared with the plasma:

    a. pH.
    b. Bicarbonate.
    c. pCO_2.
    d. Osmolarity.
    e. Glucose.

2.12   The action potential that is responsible for nerve conduction:

    a. Is an all-or-none phenomenon.
    b. Once initiated, propagates without decrement down the entire length of the nerve.
    c. Is generated by ion currents that have separate channels for Na^+ and K^+.
    d. Has a hyperpolarisation phase during which the membrane potential is even more negative than the resting phase.
    e. Requires prior hydration of the Na^+ and K^+ ions as part of the process.

2.13   The liver:

    a. Stores iron as apoferritin.
    b. Metabolises xenon.
    c. Produces alphafetoprotein in the adult.
    d. Breaks down ketone bodies to CO_2 and water.
    e. Synthesises von Willebrand factor.

2.14   Brown adipose tissue ('brown fat'):

    a. Is reduced or absent in the obese.
    b. Has a higher mitochondrial content than 'white' adipose tissue.
    c. Has a low activity level for ATP synthase.
    d. Shows more activity after eating.
    e. Is responsible for 'diet-induced thermogenesis.'

2.15 The ventricular musculature:

  a. Is a syncytium.
  b. Is an energy transducer.
  c. In its activity demonstrates the 'latch phenomenon'.
  d. Possesses both sympathetic and parasympathetic innervation in equal measure.
  e. During contraction performs as much kinetic energy work as volume-pressure work.

2.16 In the case of the heart:

  a. The resting membrane potential of its ventricular musculature is more negative than that of the sinoatrial node.
  b. It has a maximum efficiency under normal 'resting' conditions of about 66%.
  c. Atrial contraction accounts for > 50% of ventricular filling.
  d. Ventricular filling occurs mainly in mid to late diastole.
  e. Intra-atrial pressure is the same for both atria during their respective systoles.

2.17 In the case of the cardiac muscle action potential:

  a. The initial rapid depolarisation is caused by sodium movement through 'fast channels'.
  b. The plateau phase is due to activity of both Na^+ and Ca^{2+} slow channels.
  c. Activity during the plateau phase is that which is responsible for initiation of ventricular contraction.
  d. Repolarisation involves opening of K^+ channels.
  e. The refractory period is due to voltage inactivation solely of Na^+ channels.

2.18 In the case of the heart:

  a. Its energy substrate is predominantly glucose.
  b. It has a higher blood flow per unit mass than does the brain.
  c. It has a lower oxygen consumption per unit mass than the kidneys.
  d. Its parasympathetic innervation is essentially confined to the atria and their associated structures.
  e. Its venous drainage is solely via the coronary sinus.

2.19 The cardiac baroreceptor reflexes:

  a. Provide a positive feedback mechanism.
  b. Have their sensors in the carotid and aortic bodies.
  c. Have their centre in the nucleus ambiguous in the medulla.
  d. Have the vagus nerve as their sole afferent pathway.
  e. Are capable of the same intensity of activity at all blood pressure levels.

2.20 The atrioventricular node:

 a. Is situated in the right atrium just anterior to the tricuspid valve.
 b. Is innervated by the right vagus nerve.
 c. Has the lowest conduction velocity of all cardiac conducting tissues.
 d. Has fewer gap junctions than the rest of the cardiac tissues.
 e. In its healthy state does not permit retrograde conduction of impulses.

2.21 The Cardiac Index:

 a. Is a dimensionless entity.
 b. Has a normal wide range in the adult population.
 c. Progressively increases from infancy to adolescence.
 d. Increases faster with heart rate in adults compared with children.
 e. Does not usually show change until there is significant ventricular impairment.

2.22 The pulmonary endothelium:

 a. Converts angiotensin I into angiotensin II.
 b. Removes most of the bradykinin passing through it.
 c. Inactivates circulating adrenaline.
 d. Releases prostacyclin into the bloodstream.
 e. Is a source of NO for purposes of generalised systemic effects.

2.23 Concerning the right atrium:

 a. It is at the level of the carina.
 b. It is the zero reference point for arterial blood pressure measurement.
 c. It is the 'phlebostatic' point for central venous pressure determination.
 d. When full it holds more blood than the full right ventricle.
 e. Its contraction is an essential prerequisite for adequate right ventricular filling.

2.24 When measuring blood pressure by the auscultatory method and using a mercury sphygmomanometer:

 a. The (zero) reference point of the manometer must be at the level of the arm cuff.
 b. The slower the heart rate the less the error in the reading.
 c. A faster rate of cuff deflation will give a higher systolic pressure.
 d. It suffices to have a cuff bladder with a width just equal to the arm diameter.
 e. More accurate values are likely if a cuff with a single connecting tube is used.

2.25 The Na⁺–K⁺–ATPase pump:

a. Is an 'ion pump'.
b. Is present in the body in multiple isoforms.
c. Is the only primary active transport process in the body for sodium.
d. Is the sole primary active transporter in the body for potassium.
e. Is necessary for countering the passive processes arising from the Gibbs–Donnan effect.

2.26 Glucose re-absorption in the kidney:

a. Occurs almost entirely in the proximal tubule.
b. Is a primary active process.
c. Is a transcellular process.
d. At the luminal surface of the cell occurs by a process similar to that in the intestine.
e. Occurs as a counter-transport process.

2.27 The following are differences between adrenaline and noradrenaline:

a. Noradrenaline is essentially an α-agonist while adrenaline is both an α- and β-agonist.
b. Adrenaline is secreted in greater amounts by the adrenal medulla than is noradrenaline.
c. Adrenaline is removed during its passage through the pulmonary circulation, noradrenaline is not.
d. Noradrenaline increases skeletal muscle vessel blood flow. Adrenaline does not.
e. Adrenaline is metabolised by both MAO and COMT, noradrenaline by only MAO.

2.28 Ephedrine:

a. Is both an α-agonist and a β-agonist.
b. Acts both by increasing the release of endogenous noradrenaline at sympathetic endings and also by a direct action at adrenergic receptors in its own right.
c. Is metabolised by both MAO and COMT.
d. Is effective when administered enterally as well as parenterally.
e. Is available for administration as a pure isomer as well as a racemic mixture.

2.29 Concerning the enteric nervous system component of the autonomic nervous system:

a. It is derived from the neural crest.
b. Its transmitter is usually adrenaline and noradrenaline.
c. Its reflexes can be abolished by nicotinic antagonists.
d. Nitric oxide is a recognised transmitter in it.
e. It is the primary mechanism for control of alimentary tract sphincters.

2.30 During normal quiet spontaneous ventilation the work of breathing:

a. Is performed solely by the muscles of inspiration.
b. Accounts for about 5–10% of resting energy consumption.
c. Is associated with a high level of 'efficiency' of the respiratory musculature.
d. Dissipates its heat energy solely in the expiratory phase.
e. In the standard adult is minimal at a ventilation rate of about 20–25 per minute.

2.31 The following are useful tests of ventilatory capacity:

a. Maximum breathing capacity (maximum ventilation volume).
b. FEV_1.
c. Peak expiratory flow rate.
d. Vital capacity.
e. FEV_1/VC ratio.

2.32 The following are increased in concentration in the brain with an increase in normal neuronal activity:

a. Nitric oxide.
b. Lactate.
c. Adenosine.
d. Vasoactive intestinal peptide.
e. Calcitonin gene-related peptide.

2.33 Cerebral neuronal damage from ischaemia:

a. Is associated with water ingress into the neuronal cells.
b. Is accompanied by transfer of intracellular calcium from the cytosol into the endoplasmic reticulum.
c. Is ameliorated by an increase in blood glucose above its pre-ischaemic level.
d. Leads to cell membrane injury from lipid peroxidation.
e. Is associated with both cell necrosis and cell apoptosis.

2.34   Glycine receptors:

   a. Are ionotropic receptors.
   b. Are excitatory receptors.
   c. Mediate rapid synaptic transmission.
   d. Are found in the spinal cord.
   e. Are homomers.

2.35   In the convention for denoting SI units:

   a. The indicial notation ought to be preferred to the solidus notation.
   b. A capital (upper case) letter ought to be the initiating letter when writing out the full name of a unit named after a person.
   c. The abbreviated units shall have no plural form.
   d. When abbreviated, no punctuation marks viz. a full stop '.' shall be used, e.g. 1 kilogram shall be written '1 kg', not '1 kg.'.
   e. A degree sign (°) shall be used when expressing temperature in kelvin units.

2.36   The following are dimensionless entities, i.e. they are mere ratios, percentages or fractions and possess no attached units:

   a. Loschmidt number.
   b. Boltzmann constant.
   c. Sieving coefficient.
   d. Blood-gas partition coefficient.
   e. Michaelis constant.

2.37   The following are colligative properties:

   a. Osmolarity.
   b. Freezing point.
   c. Boiling point.
   d. Specific density.
   e. Vapour pressure.

2.38   The following are graded according to French catheter gauge (FCG):

   a. Carlens double lumen tube.
   b. Guedel airway.
   c. Robertshaw double lumen tube.
   d. Brain laryngeal mask airway.
   e. White double lumen tube.

2.39 The following refer to the same thing:

a. Resonant frequency and natural frequency.
b. Fluid flow rate and fluid velocity.
c. A perfect gas and an ideal gas.
d. An ideal fluid and a newtonian fluid.
e. Beer's law and Bouguer's law with respect to the propagation of light through a medium.

2.40 The amount of gas contained in each of the following cylinders can be correctly determined by applying the Ideal Gas Equation:

a. Oxygen cylinder.
b. 5% carbon dioxide in oxygen cylinder.
c. Nitrous oxide cylinder.
d. Entonox cylinder.
e. Carbon dioxide cylinder.

2.41 In the 'Fuel Cell' method of oxygen measurement:

a. There is need for an 'externally applied' potential difference.
b. The cathode is made of platinum.
c. The reaction that oxygen needs to undergo for measurement is the same as for the Clark electrode method.
d. Temperature affects the value of the readings.
e. The reading is vitiated by the presence of inhalational anaesthetic agents in the blood sample.

2.42 The term 'critical temperature' can be correctly applied to the following:

a. That temperature above which a gas cannot be liquefied by pressure alone.
b. That temperature at which a fluid's liquid and gas phases both have the same density.
c. That temperature at which a metal becomes electrically superconducting.
d. That temperature above which a ferromagnetic material loses its ferromagnetic property and becomes diamagnetic.
e. That temperature at which a gas most approximates to an ideal gas.

2.43 The 'filling ratio' of a gas cylinder:

a. Is, by definition, the weight of gas in a full cylinder divided by the weight of the liquid form of the gas occupying the whole cylinder.
b. Needs to have a lower value for cylinders in the tropics than in temperate zones.
c. Is a factor that determines the fastest rate at which a cylinder can be emptied.
d. Is relevant for a helium–oxygen cylinder.
e. Is applicable to a cyclopropane cylinder.

2.44 The following are phenomena that are relevant to magnetic resonance imaging:

a. Population inversion.
b. Precession.
c. Larmor frequency.
d. Collimation.
e. Free induction decay.

2.45 Concerning the 'Bourdon gauge' on an anaesthetic machine oxygen pathway:

a. The usefulness of its pressure reading as an indicator of amount of cylinder contents is based on the Universal Gas Equation.
b. It shows a 'linear' relationship between gauge needle and the oxygen content of the cylinder.
c. The plane of its dial-face must be inclined backwards from the vertical in accordance with International Organization for Standardization regulations.
d. Its scale showing 'low' must lie between the 6 o'clock and 9 o'clock positions of the dial-face in accordance with International Organization for Standardization regulations.
e. Its functioning principle can also be used to measure temperature.

2.46 The following will increase with a rise in temperature:

a. Solubility of a gas in a liquid.
b. MAC of an inhalational anaesthetic agent.
c. Rate of decay of a radionuclide.
d. Electrical conductivity of a semi-conductor.
e. Rate of diffusion of a gas down its concentration gradient.

2.47 In the case of the 'TEC Mark 6' Desflurane vaporiser:

a. It must be electrically energised to work correctly.
b. For the same vapour setting, it gives a lower vaporiser output for N_2O and O_2 compared with O_2 alone.
c. It has a vapour chamber capacity greater than that of conventional TEC vaporisers.
d. It has a 'closed-system' filling process.
e. It gives a higher partial pressure of the agent vapour in a hyperbaric chamber for the same concentration setting compared with that at normal atmospheric pressure.

2.48 Monopolar diathermy:

a. Necessarily requires a return electrode.
b. Necessarily requires an operational foot switch.
c. Is better for 'cutting' compared with bipolar diathermy.
d. Runs a greater risk of causing 'channelling' damage than bipolar diathermy.
e. Presently is the only satisfactory mode of diathermy available for the operation of transurethral resection of prostate.

2.49 The following inhalation anaesthetic agents are recognised as significant producers of carbon monoxide with soda lime:

a. Halothane.
b. Enflurane.
c. Isoflurane.
d. Sevoflurane.
e. Desflurane.

2.50 The production of carbon monoxide in a low flow breathing attachment with provision for CO_2 is more likely:

a. If the soda lime is dry rather than moist.
b. If potassium hydroxide (KOH) is present rather than absent.
c. If desflurane is used rather than isoflurane.
d. If the temperature of the soda lime is lower rather than higher.
e. If a zeolite were present in rather than absent from the soda lime.

2.51 The following flow devices function on the 'constant pressure/variable orifice' principle:

a. Anaesthetic machine rotameter tube.
b. The 'wall point' oxygen flowmeter tube.
c. Pitot tube.
d. Wright respirometer.
e. Ventimask.

2.52 The following are dimensionless, i.e. they are mere ratios, percentages or fractions and have no units attached to them:

a. Hufner constant.
b. Filtration coefficient.
c. Stefan constant.
d. Osmotic coefficient.
e. Universal Gas constant.

2.53 Adiabatic expansion:

a. Is a necessary phenomenon in the production of nitrogen by fractional distillation of air.
b. Is also known as the Joule–Kelvin effect.
c. Will render Boyle's law invalid.
d. Can occur at the Bodok seal when opening an oxygen cylinder on an anaesthetic machine.
e. Occurs at the end of a functioning cryoprobe.

2.54 The following are relevant to gas monitoring by the method of mass spectrometry:

a. Charge:mass ratio.
b. Volumes per cent estimation.
c. Cross-interference.
d. Penumbra effect.
e. Pressure broadening.

2.55 When the following breathing attachments are in use as indicated they must have an operational adjustable pressure-limiting (APL) valve:

a. Magill attachment during spontaneous ventilation.
b. Bain attachment during manual artificial ventilation ('hand bagging').
c. Ayre's T-piece breathing attachment with Jackson Rees modification during spontaneous paediatric ventilation.
d. Waters' to-and-fro attachment during 'hand bagging'.
e. During use of a circle breathing attachment with low fresh gas flows and mechanical artificial ventilation with a Penlon AV 900 ventilator.

2.56 Enflurane:

a. Is a chiral agent.
b. Is a stereo-isomer of isoflurane.
c. Is reputed to produce cerebral spikes.
d. On reaction with soda lime produces bromochlorodifluoroethylene (BCDFE).
e. Undergoes biotransformation to a greater extent than desflurane.

2.57 As a general rule, the 'intermediate chain' part of the structure of local anaesthetics is responsible for the following:

    a. Lipid solubility.
    b. Anaesthetic potency.
    c. Protein-binding capacity.
    d. Duration of action.
    e. Allergenicity.

2.58 Compared with bupivacaine, Lidocaine (lignocaine):

    a. Is an achiral agent.
    b. Is more extensively bound to plasma proteins.
    c. Has less CNS toxicity.
    d. Has a more rapid onset of action.
    e. Has a shorter duration of action.

2.59 The following are examples of competitive antagonism in relation to drug action:

    a. Reversal of the muscarinic effects of neostigmine with glycopyrrolate.
    b. Reversal of hypoglycaemic effect of insulin with glucagon.
    c. Reversal of the symptoms of hay fever (histamine) with H_1 receptor antagonists.
    d. Blocking of gastric acid secretion with ranitidine.
    e. Use of phenoxybenzamine to block the hypertension of phaeochromocytoma.

2.60 The following are attributes common to simple diffusion and facilitated diffusion:

    a. Neither of them requires 'extraneous' energy.
    b. Neither can occur against a concentration gradient.
    c. Neither requires a carrier protein.
    d. Neither is governed by particle size of 'transferee'.
    e. They are both temperature dependent.

2.61 The following are examples of facilitated diffusion:

    a. Movement of water across membranes through aquaporin channels.
    b. Exchange of red cell bicarbonate for plasma chloride as part of the Hamburger phenomenon.
    c. Movement of glucose from the intestinal cells into the blood capillaries.
    d. Movement of amino acids from the renal tubular lumen into the renal epithelial cell.
    e. Ion channel movement of sodium during nerve depolarisation.

2.62   In biotransformation of drugs:

a. Phase I reactions introduce or expose a functional group on the parent compound.
b. Phase II reactions generally lead to the formation of highly polar conjugates.
c. Phase I reactions normally lead to enhancement of the agent's pharmacological activity.
d. The enzyme systems of Phase I reactions are generally located in the endoplasmic reticulum.
e. All Phase II reactions take place in the cytosol.

2.63   Heparin causes a lowering of the following:

a. Platelet count.
b. Serum aldosterone.
c. Plasma potassium.
d. Thyroxine.
e. Plasma low-density lipoproteins.

2.64   The following are anti-platelet drugs:

a. Aspirin.
b. Dipyridamole.
c. Hirudin.
d. Streptokinase.
e. Abciximab

2.65   Insulin:

a. Inactivates nitric oxide synthesis.
b. Enhances renal sodium absorption.
c. Lowers plasma amino acids.
d. Hydrolyses very low-density lipoproteins (VLDLs).
e. Increases the glucosyl valine adduct of haemoglobin A.

2.66   Glucagon:

a. Is a polypeptide with disulphide linkages.
b. Is a cardiac inotrope.
c. Relaxes intestinal smooth muscle.
d. Corrects hirsutism.
e. Releases catecholamines from the adrenal medulla.

2.67   The following tend to cause hypoglycaemia:

a. Alcohol.
b. Salicylates.
c. Oral contraceptives.
d. β-adrenergic receptor antagonists.
e. Ca^{2+} channel blockers.

2.68   Anticholinesterases:

    a. Are ionised hydrophilic molecules.
    b. Antagonise acetylcholinesterase by ionic bonding.
    c. Act without exception only on the esteratic site of
       acetylcholinesterase.
    d. Can have a direct agonist effect of their own.
    e. Inhibit plasma cholinesterase.

2.69   The following neuromuscular blocking agents undergo ester
    hydrolysis by plasma esterases:

    a. Suxamethonium.
    b. Atracurium.
    c. Mivacurium.
    d. Pancuronium.
    e. Alcuronium.

2.70   Desensitisation block at nACh receptors:

    a. Is mediated by allosteric inhibition of receptor.
    b. Is independent of the classic effect resulting from competitive
       inhibition of acetylcholine.
    c. Is producible with suxamethonium.
    d. Is an effect of nicotine.
    e. Can be produced by cocaine.

2.71   The following drugs inhibit butyrylcholinesterase:

    a. Nupercaine.
    b. Metoclopramide.
    c. Ranitidine.
    d. Bambuterol.
    e. Esmolol.

2.72   Following their release the following neurotransmitters are
    inactivated primarily by re-uptake into their respective pre-
    synaptic terminals:

    a. Acetylcholine at skeletal NMJs.
    b. Adrenaline at adrenergic nerves.
    c. Glutamate.
    d. GABA.
    e. Serotonin.

2.73 The following are agonist/antagonist opioids:

a. Buprenorphine.
b. Nalbuphine.
c. Nalorphine.
d. Naloxone.
e. Pentazocine.

2.74 The following opioids produce metabolites that have analgesic activity in their own right:

a. Alfentanil.
b. Fentanyl.
c. Morphine.
d. Pethidine.
e. Remifentanil.

2.75 The muscle rigidity seen with opioid analgesics:

a. Is confined to piperidine derivatives.
b. Is limited to the trunk.
c. Is more commonly seen at emergence from anaesthesia than at induction.
d. Is chiefly manifest as severe reduction of chest wall compliance.
e. Is reversible with naloxone.

2.76 Adenosine:

a. Has a half-life of the order of seconds rather than minutes.
b. Decreases coronary blood flow.
c. Increases cellular oxygen consumption.
d. Slows AV conduction by reducing Ca^{2+} conductance.
e. Converts atrial fibrillation and atrial flutter to sinus rhythm.

2.77 Of the IV anaesthetic agents thiopentone, methohexitone, propofol, etomidate and ketamine:

a. Propofol is the only one that is not presented for use as a racemic mixture.
b. Ketamine is the only one that increases $CMRO_2$.
c. Thiopentone is the only one that contains sulphur.
d. Methohexitone is the only one that is an anti-analgesic.
e. Etomidate is the only one that has been associated with haemolysis.

2.78   Thiopentone:

a. Is presented for use as a markedly alkaline solution.
b. Has a pKa comparable with that of the plasma.
c. Manifests tautomerism, i.e. dynamic isomerism.
d. Shows marked changes in its degree of ionisation with small variations of environmental pH.
e. On IV injection shows significant uptake in the lungs.

2.79   In equi-anaesthetic dosage, propofol:

a. Is a more potent depressor of laryngeal reflexes than thiopentone.
b. Is a more potent bronchodilator than halothane.
c. Is a more potent peripheral vasodilator than etomidate.
d. Is a more potent skeletal muscle relaxant than di-ethyl ether.
e. Has a greater anti-analgesic action than methohexitone.

2.80   Unpleasant emergence reactions after ketamine anaesthesia include:

a. Vivid dreaming.
b. Extracorporeal experiences (sense of floating out of one's body).
c. Illusions.
d. Uncontrolled vocalisations.
e. Sense of severe depression.

2.81   The following are additives present in benzodiazepine preparations:

a. Sodium benzoate.
b. Di-sodium edetate.
c. Sodium carbonate.
d. Sodium bicarbonate.
e. Sodium hydroxide.

2.82   Concerning hypoxic pulmonary vasoconstriction:

a. The phenomenon is present predominantly in the arteriolar segments of the pulmonary vasculature.
b. The primary oxygen sensor is in the pulmonary endothelium.
c. Voltage-sensitive potassium (K_V) channels are an essential pre-requisite for its occurrence.
d. It is a phenomenon absent from the fetal lung circulation.
e. It is attenuated by ET-1.

2.83 **Aspirin:**

   a. Inactivates cyclo-oxygenase as well as lipoxygenase.
   b. Inhibits COX 1 as well as COX 2.
   c. Can increase bleeding both by altering platelet adhesiveness and by causing hypocoagulability.
   d. Can cause both a respiratory acidosis as well as a metabolic acidosis.
   e. Can raise body temperature as well as lower body temperature.

2.84 **In the management of paracetamol poisoning there is a place for:**

   a. Gastric lavage.
   b. Forced diuresis.
   c. Renal dialysis.
   d. Infusion of sulphur-containing amino acids.
   e. Administration of vitamin K.

2.85 **Diclofenac:**

   a. Is a chiral agent.
   b. Is chemically an acid.
   c. Is a non-specific COX inhibitor.
   d. Produces methaemoglobinaemia as a side effect.
   e. Is excreted predominantly unchanged in the urine.

2.86 **Compared with nitrous oxide, xenon has a:**

   a. Lower blood-gas partition coefficient.
   b. Higher MAC.
   c. Greater tendency to cause pulmonary hypertension.
   d. Higher oil-gas partition coefficient.
   e. Lower degree of biotransformation.

2.87 **The following are higher in a neonate compared with a standard young adult:**

   a. Anatomical dead space volume per kg body weight.
   b. Daily loss of body water as a percentage of total body water.
   c. Body surface area per unit body weight.
   d. Heat loss from head as a percentage of whole-body heat loss.
   e. Blood volume per kg body weight.

2.88 **Hypotension in the immediate postoperative phase (i.e. in the Recovery ward) is a likely occurrence:**

a. If the patient is moderately hypercapnic.
b. If the patient shows signs of confusion.
c. If patient complains of angina.
d. Where the patient is nauseated.
e. If the patient shows signs of respiratory difficulty.

2.89 **In a spontaneously breathing patient under general anaesthesia:**

a. Chest movement is an accurate indicator of effective ventilation.
b. The degree of movement of the 'breathing' bag is an adequate index of the tidal volume.
c. An SpO_2 in the upper 90s is proof of adequate alveolar ventilation.
d. Near normocapnia is an accurate index of the adequacy of ventilation.
e. The presence of peripheral cyanosis necessarily indicates alveolar hypoxia.

2.90 **In myasthenia gravis, the muscle weakness:**

a. Is commonly in the distal musculature.
b. Is associated with pain.
c. In the female is worst during the mid-menstrual phase.
d. Is associated with muscle wasting.
e. Is associated with a loss of tendon reflexes.

2.1 Answers

a. **True**.
b. **True**.
c. **False** – right atrium.
d. **True**.
e. **False** – by the left vagus.

2.2 Answers

a. **True**.
b. **True**.
c. **False** – the genital branch is the motor supply to the cremaster muscle and is the nervous pathway involved in the cremasteric reflex. The femoral branch of the genitofemoral nerve is entirely cutaneous and sensory.
d. **True**.
e. **True**.

2.3 Answers

a. **False** – the facial nerve has no cutaneous distribution.
b. **True** – the maxillary nerve supplies the lower eyelid, cheek, side of nose and skin (and mucous membrane) of the upper lip.
c. **False** – the first cervical nerve has no cutaneous distribution.
d. **False** – the spinal part of the accessory nerve is the motor supply to the sternomastoid and trapezius muscles.
e. **True** – a very small area anterior to the auricle.

2.4 Answers

a. **False** – ipsilateral enophthalmos.
b. **False** – ipsilateral hypohydrosis.
c. **False** – ipsilateral partial ptosis, because the levator palpebrae superioris muscle, which elevates the upper eye lid, has a dual nerve supply – sympathetic from the sympathetic ganglion and a branch from the oculomotor. Only the former is paralysed.
d. **True** – there is ipsilateral miosis, therefore a contralateral relative mydriasis.
e. **True** – because of loss of (sympathetic) vasoconstriction.

2.5 Answers

a. **True**.
b. **True**.
c. **False** – runs in the wall of the sinus.
d. **False** – runs in the wall of the sinus.
e. **False** – runs in the wall of the sinus.

2.6 Answers

a. **True** – but since the movement of water anywhere in the body is passive, depending on the presence of a 'gradient', it does not move into the brain cells easily because of the relative impermeability of the blood–brain barrier to sodium. See **b.** below.

b. **False** – only slightly permeable.

c. **True** – it must be, otherwise cerebral hypoxia is a certainty.

d. **True** – it must be, so as to facilitate its easy removal.

e. **True** – hence the ease with which alcohol intoxication occurs.

2.7 Answers

a. **False**.

b. **True**.

c. **True** – because both H^+ and CO_2 compete with each other for the $-NH_2$ group of the amino acids of the globin chains.

d. **False** – is antagonised by 2,3 DPG.

e. **False**.

2.8 Answers

a. **False** – Paul Bert effect – convulsions caused by oxygen toxicity.

b. **False** – Bernoulli phenomenon – law of conservation of mechanical energy as applied to fluid flow in a tube.

c. **True** – Bohr effect – rightward shift of the haemoglobin O_2 dissociation curve with a rise in pCO_2.

d. **True** – the 'chloride shift' (movement of chloride into the red cell in exchange for bicarbonate) in venous blood.

e. **False** – Fink effect – diffusion hypoxia resulting during recovery from nitrous oxide anaesthesia, when larger volumes of the agent leave the system and are replaced by smaller volumes of nitrogen. This leads to a higher percentage of alveolar N_2O and consequently a lower alveolar FiO_2, and therefore hypoxia.

2.9 Answers

a. **True** – by acting at $GABA_A$-mediated synapses, but may also exert some of its effects by inhibiting NMDA receptors and potentiating $5HT_3$ receptor activity.

b. **False** – primarily but not exclusively. Ethanol also activates nitric oxide synthase leading to release of NO, which also causes vasodilatation.

c. **False** – increases the level of plasma HDLs.

d. **False** – inhibits voltage-gated L-type Ca^{2+} channels.

e. **True** – therefore extracellular adenosine concentrations rise, leading to alcohol-induced neuronal depression.

2.10 Answers

a. **True**.
b. **True**.
c. **False**.
d. **True** – metoclopramide enhances gastric emptying and thus increases intestinal absorption of alcohol.
e. **True** – (i) alcohol is poorly absorbed by fat. Women have more subcutaneous fat and a smaller blood volume and therefore blood and non-fat tissue concentrations are higher; and (ii) women have lower concentrations of alcohol dehydrogenase, especially in the gastric mucosal cells.

2.11 Answers

a. **False** – pH 7.33; plasma pH 7.40.
b. **False** – about the same.
c. **True** – c. 50 mmHg c. 6.7 kPa; plasma CO_2 c. 40 mmHg; c. 5.3 kPa.
d. **False** – about the same: c. 290 mosmol/L.
e. **False** – c. 3.5–4 mmol/L; plasma glucose c. 4–5.5/L.

2.12 Answers

a. **True**.
b. **True**.
c. **True**.
d. **True**.
e. **False** – quite the opposite. The Na^+ and K^+ ions must have their attached water molecules removed to make them small enough to pass through the channels.

2.13 Answers

a. **False** – stores it as ferritin. Apoferritin is the protein to which the iron is bound.
b. **False** – xenon is exhaled unchanged.
c. **False** – alphafetoprotein is almost totally replaced by albumin by the end of the first year of life.
d. **False** – the liver is the only organ that does not contain ketoacyl CoA transferase (also known as acetoacetate – succinyl CoA transferase), an enzyme required for the breakdown of ketone bodies.
e. **False** – von Willebrand factor, a glycoprotein, is not produced by the liver, but by vascular endothelial cells and megakaryocytes.

2.14 Answers

a. **True**.
b. **True**.
c. **True** – therefore there is less ATP, and therefore less free energy that is convertible to fat is trapped in it.
d. **True**.
e. **True** – it can be active in normal individuals, which accounts for their ability to 'eat and not get fat'.

2.15 Answers

a. **True** – this is due to the presence of 'gap junctions', which allow free diffusion of ions and therefore rapid conduction of the action potential across the musculature.
b. **True** – it converts chemical energy into mechanical energy. A tranducer is a device that converts one form of energy into another.
c. **False** – 'latch phenomenon' – the continued maintenance of full contraction with a level of activity much less than that which was required to attain that full contraction, by utilising a level of energy equal to a fraction of that which was initially required for full contraction. It is an attribute of smooth muscle.
d. **False** – there is very little parasympathetic supply, if at all, to the ventricles.
e. **False** – nearly 99% of the energy expenditure is to perform volume-pressure work. Only c.1% is for kinetic work.

2.16 Answers

a. **True** – sinoatrial node –55 to –60 mV; ventricular muscle fibre –85 to –90 mV.
b. **False** – maximum efficiency c. 20–25%. 'Efficiency' – ratio of (mechanical) energy output to (chemical) energy input.
c. **False** – atrial contraction normally accounts for only c. 25% of ventricular filling. This is why patients with atrial fibrillation continue to have a reasonable cardiac output, unless they are tachycardic.
d. **False** – first third of diastole – period of rapid ventricular filling. Third third of diastole – atrial contraction leading to 25% of ventricular filling. See **c**.
e. **False** – right atrium: 4–6 mmHg; left atrium: 7–8 mmHg.

2.17 Answers

a. **True**.
b. **True**.
c. **True**.
d. **True**.
e. **False** – both Na^+ and K^+ channels.

2.18 Answers

a. **False** – the heart's main energy substrate is long chain fatty acids such as palmitate, triglycerides. It does also utilise glucose, ketones and to a small extent amino acids.

b. **True** – brain: c. 55 ml per 100 g tissue; heart: c. 75 ml per 100 g tissue.

c. **False** – higher. Heart: c. 8.5 ml; kidneys: c. 7 ml/100 g tissue.

d. **True**.

e. **False** – some blood drains directly into all four chambers of the heart through minute thebesian veins.

2.19 Answers

a. **False** – negative feedback mechanism – a rise in blood pressure leads to inhibition of centres, leading to a fall in heart rate and to reflex vasodilatation.

b. **False** – in the carotid and aortic sinuses. The 'bodies' are chemoreceptors.

c. **False** – the nucleus solitarius. The nucleus ambiguous is a motor nucleus.

d. **False** – the vagus is the afferent pathway from the aortic sinus, the glossopharyngeal nerve from the carotid sinus.

e. **False** – the baroreceptors lose their functional capacity at pressures below about 50 mmHg.

2.20 Answers

a. **False** – is situated just posterior to the tricuspid valve.

b. **False** – its predominant innervation is by the left vagus nerve.

c. **True** – the aim is to delay conduction to the ventricles so as to allow for full emptying of atrial blood into the ventricles prior to commencement of ventricular systole.

d. **True** – for the reasons stated in **c**.

e. **True** – it is the only cardiac tissue that does not permit retrograde conduction under normal conditions.

2.21 Answers

a. **False** – The Cardiac Index is the cardiac output per unit body surface area, and therefore its units are: litres per minute per square metre.

b. **False** – its range is fairly narrow.

c. **True** – neonate c. 2.5L/min/m^2; 2-year-old c. 3.0; 5-year-old c. 3.7; 12-year-old c. 4.3.

d. **True**.

e. **True** – it is therefore a relatively insensitive index of ventricular performance.

2.22 Answers

a. **True** – because it contains ACE.
b. **True** – to the extent of 80%.
c. **False** – adrenaline is not removed (nor is histamine or dopamine) but noradrenaline is.
d. **True** – by synthesising it from endogenous arachidonic acid in the lung.
e. **False** – although the lung endothelium secretes NO its intended effect is local vasodilatation. NO is rapidly inactivated by haemoglobin and therefore cannot exert a generalised systemic effect.

2.23 Answers

a. **False** – the carina is about one vertebral body thickness above the right atrium.
b. **True**.
c. **True** – the phlebostatic point is the reference point for CVP measurement. It is the point of decussation of the phlebostatic axis (a horizontal line in the midaxilla in a supine subject) and a vertical line passing down from the fourth intercostal space anteriorly.
d. **True** – the total blood volume of the heart when all its chambers are full is about 500–550 ml. More than half of this is in the atria, which together hold nearly 300 ml; the right atrium holds about 150 ml and the right ventricle about 120 ml.
e. **False** – 75% of right ventricular filling is 'passive', depending merely on the presence of an open tricuspid valve. Right atrial contraction contributes a mere 25% of the ventricular blood volume.

2.24 Answers

a. **False** – the zero reference point for all intravascular pressure measurements ought to be the level of the right atrium.
b. **False** – the error is greater; a lower reading is obtained.
c. **False** – lower.
d. **False** – for accuracy of measurement the width of the cuff bladder ought to be 20% more than arm diameter.
e. **False** – less accurate, because of the pressure drop along the tube during cuff deflation.

2.25 Answers

a. **True** – in fact it was the first to be recognised as an ion pump, earning its discoverer, Jens Skou, the Nobel Prize for Chemistry in 1997.
b. **True** – there are at least four α-subunit and two β-subunit isoforms.
c. **True**.
d. **False**.
e. **True**.

2.26 Answers

a. **True** – 98% of glucose is absorbed in the proximal tubule.
b. **False** – glucose absorption is essentially a secondary active transport process, depending on the concurrent movement of sodium down a concentration gradient and aided by a SGLT.
c. **True**.
d. **True**.
e. **False** – it is part of a co-transport process because the sodium (the 'co-transportee') moves in the same direction as the glucose.

2.27 Answers

a. **True**.
b. **True** – adrenaline c. 80%; noradrenaline c. 20%.
c. **False** – it's the other way round – 25% of noradrenaline is removed, adrenaline is not.
d. **False** – adrenaline, being a β-agonist, dilates skeletal muscle vessels, noradrenaline does not.
e. **False** – both adrenaline and noradrenaline are metabolised by both MAO and COMT.

2.28 Answers

a. **True** – it increases the heart rate and force of myocardial contraction and also the peripheral resistance.
b. **True**.
c. **False** – it is metabolised by neither. The absence of –OH groups at positions 3 and 4 on the benzene ring makes ephedrine immune from breakdown by COMT, and the presence of a –CH_3 group on the α carbon atom of the ethylamine moiety blocks oxidation by MAO.
d. **True** – because of resistance to metabolism by COMT (see **c**).
e. **True** – ephedrine has two chiral carbon atoms and therefore has four isomers: *d*- and *l*-ephedrine and *d*- and *l*-pseudoephedrine. *l*-ephedrine is the more potent isomer. The racemic mixture is also available for clinical use.

2.29 Answers

a. **True** – from the neuroblasts of the neural crest.
b. **False** – the transmitter is predominantly acetylcholine.
c. **True**.
d. **True**.
e. **False** – this function is provided by the sympathetic and parasympathetic systems.

2.30 Answers

a. **True** – expiration is a purely passive process dependent on the elastic recoil of the lungs and chest wall utilising the potential energy stored in them during inspiration.
b. **False** – c. 1–2%.
c. **False** – low level of efficiency, viz. c.10%. 'efficiency' = work output as a percentage of energy input. cf. petrol consumption of a motor car – miles per gallon.
d. **False** – about half the heat loss is produced (and dissipated) in the inspiratory phase in overcoming the frictional forces opposing inspiration.
e. **False** – minimal at a rate of c. 15 per minute, because at this rate of ventilation both the work done in overcoming elastic recoil of the lungs and that in overcoming airway and tissue resistance are minimal.

2.31 Answers

a. **True**.
b. **True**.
c. **True**.
d. **False**.
e. **False** – indicates airway resistance.

2.32 Answers

a. **True**.
b. **True**.
c. **True**.
d. **True**.
e. **True**.

2.33 Answers

a. **True** – because of loss of activity of Na^+–K^+–ATPase pump.
b. **False** – Ca is transferred from the ER to the cytosol.
c. **False** – is worsened by a rise in blood glucose because anaerobic glycolysis leads to an acidosis, which is detrimental to neuronal integrity.
d. **True** – because of the release of free radicals.
e. **True**.

2.34 Answers

a. **True**.
b. **False** – inhibitory receptors.
c. **True**.
d. **True**.
e. **True** – they contain only α subunits, unlike GABA receptors, which function only as heteromers.

2.35 Answers

a. **True** – e.g. m s^{-2}, not m/s^2.
b. **False** – but a capital letter must be used when used as an abbreviation, e.g. 'A' when indicating 'ampere'.
c. **True** – e.g. 500 metres is written '500 m', not '500 ms'. ('ms' denotes 'milliseconds').
d. **True**.
e. **False** – the kelvin scale is an absolute temperature scale and therefore there can be no 'degrees' of kelvin.

2.36 Answers

a. **False** – Loschmidt number – the number of particles per unit volume of an ideal gas at STP – x per metre^3. Therefore it has a unit, i.e. 'metre^{-3}'. It is 2.68×10^{25} per cubic metre. It was named after Joseph Loschmidt (1821–1895). (Note – Avogadro's number is the number of particles per gram mole of the gas and is 6.02×10^{23}).
b. **False** – ratio of the Universal Gas constant to the Avogadro constant and is equal to c. 1.38×10^{-23} joules per kelvin. It may be regarded as the gas constant per molecule.
c. **True** – the sieving coefficient is to a solute what the (renal) filtration coefficient is to plasma. It is the ratio of solute concentration in the glomerular ultrafiltrate to that in the plasma.
d. **True** – the ratio at equilibrium in which an agent will distribute itself between two compartments of equal volume separated by a membrane to which the agent is permeable.
e. **False** – Michaelis constant K_m. – the concentration of a substrate in mol per unit volume required in order for an enzyme to act at half its maximum velocity (V_{max}) in an enzyme-controlled reaction.

2.37 Answers

All are **true** except **d**. A colligative property is one that depends solely on the number of particles of the agent and not on their size, mass, charge or chemistry. The 'specific density' is the mass per unit volume.

2.38 Answers

a. **True** – Carlens tubes are of sizes 35, 37, 39 and 41.
b. **False** – graded as – 000, 00, 0, 1, 2, 3 and 4.
c. **False** – graded as small, medium and large.
d. **False** – numbered as 1, 2, 3, 4 and 5.
e. **True** – the White tube is a right-sided Carlens tube and therefore is graded as the Carlens tube. Note: Carlens did not design a right-sided tube (contrast Robertshaw), as he was a physician who used his tube to test lung function by bronchospirometry in conscious patients, placing the tube in the tracheobronchial tract under local anaesthesia! FCG is a unit with dimensions. It is the external circumference of the device in millimetres. Steel wire gauge (SWG) has no dimensions; it refers to the number of the particular device that can be accommodated in a standard measuring device. For this reason the higher the SWG number, the smaller the bore of the device, e.g. cannulae.

2.39 Answers

a. **True**.
b. **False** – fluid flow rate is the volume of fluid passing a point per unit time. Fluid velocity is the speed at which a fluid volume passes a point.
c. **True**.
d. **False** – an ideal fluid is non-compressible; it has no internal frictional forces, i.e. viscosity. A newtonian fluid, in its flow, conforms to the Hagen–Poiseuille equation. It possesses viscosity but this does not vary with its shear rate.
e. **False** – Beer's law states that the intensity of light varies inversely with the square of the density of its medium of propagation. Bouguer's law (or Lambert's law) states that the intensity of light is inversely proportional to the distance of propagation.

2.40 Answers

a. **True**.
b. **True**.
c. **False**.
d. **True**.
e. **False**.

Note: if the agent is in entirely gaseous form then the contents can be determined by applying the Ideal Gas Equation: $PV = nRT$

The following are constant: V is the internal volume of the cylinder; R is the gas constant; T is the kelvin temperature. Therefore P (pressure of the cylinder content) is proportional to n (number of moles of the gas).

2.41 Answers

a. **False** – the fuel cell is a 'voltaic' cell and thus generates its own electrical energy.
b. **False** – it is made of gold.
c. **True** – oxygen combines with electrons to form OH^- (hydroxyl) ions.
d. **True** – the temperature of the electrolyte solution will determine the amount of oxygen in solution and therefore the eventual oxygen reading.
e. **True** – the presence of nitrous oxide affects the accuracy of measurement.

2.42 Answers

a. **True** – this is the conventional definition of 'critical temperature'.
b. **True** – this is the same as **a**.
c. **False** – this is the 'transition temperature'.
d. **False** – this is the 'Curie temperature', after Pierre Curie.
e. **False** – this is the 'Boyle temperature' of a gas, named after Robert Boyle of Boyle's law fame.

2.43 Answers

a. **False** – the ratio – weight of gas in full cylinder divided by the weight of water that can occupy the whole cylinder.
b. **False** – needs to be lower (0.65) for temperate zones than for the Tropics (0.75) because the variation in temperature round the year is greater in temperate climes.
c. **False** – not a material factor.
d. **False** – because the agent mixture is entirely in gaseous form.
e. **True** – because the contents of a 'full' cyclopropane cylinder are partly liquid.

2.44 Answers

a. **False** – population inversion is a phenomenon related to laser activity.
b. **True** – precession – the 'wobbling' of the activated protons in the applied magnetic field, like the wobble of a spinning top.
c. **True** – the frequency of precession of the protons (number of 'wobbles' per second).
d. **False** – this is a property of laser light.
e. **True** – this is a decrease in signal recorded by the receiver coil in the transverse plane when the radio frequency pulse is switched off during magnetic resonance imaging.

2.45 Answers

a. **True** – the equation is:

$$PV = nRT$$

V is the inside volume of the cylinder; R is the universal gas constant; T is the kelvin temperature. All of these are constants, therefore P is proportional to n, the number of moles, i.e. the amount of oxygen remaining in the cylinder.

b. **True**.
c. **True** – by an angle of 15 degrees.
d. **True**.
e. **True** – a change in temperature will lead to a change in the pressure of the gas in the Bourdon tube and this latter change is reflected in the movement of the gauge needle.

2.46 Answers

a. **False** – it decreases.
b. **True** – c. 2–5% per degree celsius rise in body temperature.
c. **False** – the rate of decay of a radionuclide is independent of temperature.
d. **True** – a conductor shows a fall in electrical conductance (i.e. an increase in resistance) with a rise in temperature. Semi-conductors and insulators show the opposite effect.
e. **True** – because the molecules of the gas become energetically more active with a temperature rise.

2.47 Answers

a. **True**.
b. **True** – because N_2O has a lower viscosity.
c. **True** – c. 425–450 ml, compared with 150–250 ml. This is necessary because desflurane has a high MAC compared with other common inhalational agents and therefore there has to be a bigger reservoir to accommodate more volume of the agent liquid.
d. **True** – the 'saf-T-fil' method.
e. **True**.

2.48 Answers

a. **True** – 'monopolar' means that only one 'pole' of the electrical pathway is in the surgeon's hand. Therefore there must be a return pathway for the electric current, which is provided by the return lead via the diathermy plate. (Note: even bipolar diathermy needs a return pathway, which is provided by one of the 'tines' of the surgical forceps.)

b. **False** – it does require a switch but it need not necessarily be foot operated; it can be operated with a hand-held switch.

c. **True** – it is possible to snip with bipolar current, but effective cutting requires the monopolar mode.

d. **True** – 'channelling' is the return of (part of) the diathermy current by way of a pathway (particularly an attenuated one) other than the intended one.

e. **True**.

2.49 Answers

a. **False** – halothane has been said to produce very minute amounts of CO, which is of no clinical significance.

b. **True**.

c. **True**.

d. **False**. This is the same as for halothane (see **a.**)

e. **True**.

Agents with a $-CHF_2$ moiety in their structure have a tendency to produce CO with soda lime. This is true of desflurane, enflurane and isoflurane in that order. Halothane produces bromochloro-difluoroethylene (BCDFE) with soda lime. Sevoflurane does not have a $-CHF_2$ moiety (it has a $-CFH_2$ moiety) but yet can produce CO (in minute amounts) via the Cannizzaro disproportionation reaction. The Cannizzaro reaction is named after Stanislao Cannizzaro (1826–1910), an Italian chemist. It is a reaction of aldehydes to give carboxylic acids and alcohols, and is a 'disproportionation reaction' because the same compound is reduced and oxidised. In the following example benzenecarbaldehyde is oxidised to benzenecarboxylic acid and reduced to benzene alcohol:

$$2\ C_6H_5\ CHO + H_2O = C_6H_5\ COOH + C_6H_5\ CH_2OH$$

2.50 Answers

a. **True**.
b. **True**.
c. **True** – inhalational anaesthetic agents with the $-CHF_2$ moiety in their chemical structure produce CO with soda lime. Both desflurane and isoflurane (as well as enflurane) produce CO – desflurane > enflurane > isoflurane. Sevoflurane does not have a $-CHF_2$ moiety (it has a CFH_2 moiety) but yet can produce CO via the 'cannizarro disproportionation reaction'.
d. **False** – higher temperatures, especially by drying out the soda lime, are more likely to cause CO production.
e. **False** – zeolites help retain moisture and could help reduce the likelihood of CO production.

2.51 Answers

a. **True**.
b. **True**.
c. **False** – The Pitot tube is a 'constant orifice, differential pressure' device.
d. **False**.
e. **False**.

2.52 Answers

a. **False** – the combining power of O_2 with Hb, which is (1.34) ml per gram.
b. **True** – usually applied to glomerular filtration, the filtration coefficient is the glomerular filtrate (c. 120 ml per minute) as a fraction of the renal plasma flow (c. 600 ml per minute) and is therefore c. 20%.
c. **False** – The Stefan constant is joules per K^4. It is the proportionality constant s in the The Stefan–Boltzmann equation, $E = s \times T^4$, i.e. the energy of electromagnetic radiations E. is proportional to the fourth power of their kelvin temperature. The Stefan–Boltzmann equation is the basis of the working principle of the infra-red thermometer.
d. **True** – the osmotic coefficient is a measure of the extent to which an electrolyte is dissociated into its constituent ions when in solution and therefore is expressed as a percentage or a fraction. For a fully dissociated electrolyte the osmotic coefficient is 1.0.
e. **False** – R is joules per kelvin per mole.

2.53 Answers

a. **True**.

b. **True** – or the Joule–Thomson effect, because Sir William Thomson became Lord Kelvin.

c. **True** – because Boyle's law holds good only under isothermal (and not adiabatic) conditions.

d. **False** – at a Bodok seal there is adiabatic compression.

e. **True**.

2.54 Answers

a. **True** – in mass spectrometry the amount of a gas present is determined by the degree of deflection of the ions of the gas in accordance with the mass:charge ratio. The higher the charge:mass ratio (or the lower the mass:charge ratio), the greater the degree of deflection of the ions and therefore the higher the concentration of the agent in the gas mixture.

b. **True** – mass spectrometry estimates gases according to volumes per cent in the mixture of gases and not according to partial pressure.

c. **True** – if similar agents are present there may be overlap of the beams of deflection of the different agents.

d. **False** – penumbra effect is a phenomenon of pulse oximetry, when some of the light from the LED reaches the photodetector without passing through the tissue bed, a more likely occurrence in patients with strong pulsations.

e. **False** – pressure broadening is a phenomenon observed with infra-red gas analysis methods. Changes in the total pressure of a gas mixture will affect the width of the infra-red absorption bands of individual gases in the mixture. For instance, as the pressure of the gas mixture increases, the presence of oxygen, although oxygen is not amenable to analysis by this method, will nevertheless make the CO_2 absorption bands narrower. On the other hand, the presence of N_2O will cause broadening of the absorption bands of CO_2.

2.55 Answers

a. **True**.

b. **True** – the valve needs to be partially closed, but nevertheless needs to be operational.

c. **False** – when using an Ayre's T-piece attachment for paediatric anaesthesia there are no valves incorporated into the system.

d. **True** – like in **b** above, the valve needs to be partially closed yet operational.

e. **False** – during mechanical ventilation that part of the attachment incorporating the APL valve is bypassed and is therefore non-operational.

2.56 Answers

a. **True** – of the currently available inhalational anaesthetic agents sevoflurane is the only one that is achiral.
b. **False** – it is a structural isomer of isoflurane.
c. **True** – seizure-type discharges have been recorded during enflurane anaesthesia.
d. **False** – it is halothane that produces BCDFE.
e. **True** – c. 2–2.5% compared with desflurane 0.02%.

2.57 Answers

a. **False** – lipid solubility is a property of the aromatic side moiety.
b. **True** – the greater the length of the 'intermediate chain' (and the side amino group), the greater the potency (and the toxicity) of the agent.
c. **True** – protein binding is a particular property of the amide LAs. The amide moiety is the 'intermediate chain' of amide LAs.
d. **False** – owes it to the hydrophobic aromatic moiety.
e. **True** – the amide LAs are more likely to cause allergic reactions.

2.58 Answers

a. **True** – bupivacaine is a chiral agent, lignocaine is achiral.
b. **False** – lignocaine: c. 70%, bupivacaine: c. 95%.
c. **True** – ratio of CNS toxicity – lidocaine – bupivacaine: – 1 – 4.
d. **True** – because its pK_a is 7.7 and thus nearer to the extracellular pH (7.4) than bupivacaine, which has a pK_a of 8.1.
e. **True**.

2.59 Answers

a. **True**.
b. **False** – physiological antagonism.
c. **True**.
d. **True**.
e. **False** – non-competitive (pharmacological) antagonism.

Note: drug antagonism may be:

1. Pharmacological – here the antagonist prevents an agonist from interacting with its receptors to produce an effect. The type of antagonism can be *competitive* or *non-competitive*. Competitive antagonists compete with agonists in a reversible fashion for the same receptor site, (e.g. **a**. above). Non-competitive antagonists bind irreversibly to the receptor site or another site that inhibits the response to the agonist. No matter how much agonist is given, the action of the agonist cannot be overcome, (e.g. **e**. above).

2. Physiological – here the antagonism is to the physiological effect of the agonist and is brought about by the antagonist acting at a *different* receptor. For example, the reversal of the hypotensive effect of a spinal or epidural (resulting from blockade at the sympathetic ganglia) by the administration of a vasoconstrictor, e.g. metaraminol, which acts on the peripheral vasomotor receptor sites (α_1-adrenergic receptor).

3. Chemical (also called antagonism by neutralisation) – occurs when the 'agonist' and the 'antagonist' combine chemically to form a neutral compound. Examples of this are as follows: (i) heparin reversal by protamine; (ii) neutralisation of gastric acid by oral citrate.

2.60 Answers

a. **True**.
b. **True**.
c. **False** – facilitated diffusion requires a carrier protein.
d. **False** – according to Graham's law of diffusion, the rate of simple diffusion of a substance is inversely proportional to the square root of its molecular weight.
e. **True** – in the case of facilitated diffusion, temperature will determine the activity of the carrier protein. In simple diffusion, temperature will determine the 'intrinsic' energy and therefore the activity of the diffusing substance, and therefore the rate of diffusion.

2.61 Answers

a. **False** – facilitated diffusion is a *carrier*-mediated transport process. Water transport is essentialy a *channel*-mediated process, the channel in this case being aquaporin.

b. **True** – the two ions, bicarbonate and chloride, share the same transfer protein, although travelling in opposite directions – countertransport.

c. **True** – using the carrier protein GLUT 1.

d. **True** – the mechanism is the same as in **c**.

e. **False** – movement of Na^+ (and K^+) during nerve impulse transmission occurs by passive transport through voltage-gated ion channels, aqueous pores which are highly selective for the particular ions and which open and close on receipt of a signal. Since they are not dependent on carrier proteins but merely on a concentration gradient and an open gate, their movement is much faster than that of the Na^+–K^+–ATPase pump. This is clearly necessary in particular for impulse transmission in nerves, which need to be very rapid.

2.62 Answers

a. **True**.

b. **True** – so that they may be excreted more easily via the kidney.

c. **False** – Phase I reactions usually, though not necessarily, convert drugs to inactive metabolites.

d. **True**.

e. **False** – glucuronide conjugation, a Phase II reaction, usually takes place in the endoplasmic reticulum.

2.63 Answers

a. **True**.

b. **True**.

c. **False** – it causes hyperkalaemia, which may be secondary to the lowering of aldosterone. See **b**.

d. **False** – it raises it.

e. **True**.

2.64 Answers

a. **True** – affects platelet activity by covalent acetylation of serine moieties near the active site of cyclo-oxygenase.

b. **True** – interferes with platelet function by increasing intracellular cAMP.

c. **False** – prolongs coagulation by binding to and inactivating thrombin.

d. **False** – acts as a fibrinolysin.

e. **True**.

2.65 Answers

a. False – insulin activates NO synthesis.
b. True.
c. True – by converting them into protein.
d. True – insulin hydrolyses triglycerides present in VLDLs, releasing IDLs, which are then converted in the liver to the more cholesterol-rich LDLs.
e. True – this is the basis of the HbA_{1c} estimation in diabetes.

2.66 Answers

a. False – it is a polypeptide but it has no disulphide bonds, compare insulin.
b. True – glucagon is a positive cardiac inotrope (and chronotrope).
c. True.
d. False – it is metformin, a biguanide antidiabetic agent that corrects hirsutism.
e. True – it has been used as a test for phaeochromocytoma.

2.67 Answers

a. True – by inhibiting gluconeogenesis.
b. True – (i) by enhancing pancreatic β-cell sensitivity to glucose and thereby promoting insulin secretion; and (ii) by a weak peripheral insulin-like action on tissues.
c. False – OCPs have a direct effect on peripheral tissues, which counteracts insulin action.
d. True – (i) inhibit catecholamine action of gluconeogenesis; and (ii) mask the symptoms of a fall in blood sugar caused by insulin such as tremors and palpitations.
e. False – these cause hyperglycaemia by direct inhibition of insulin secretion.

2.68 Answers

a. True.
b. False – by covalent bonding, except for edrophonium, which does so by electrostatic actions between the agent and acetylcholinesterase.
c. False – most act only on the esteratic site, but edrophonium acts at the anionic site as well as the esteratic site.
d. True.
e. True.

2.69 Answers

a. **True** – butyrylcholinesterase.
b. **True** – atracurium is broken down mainly by Hofmann degradation, but plasma esterase breakdown also plays a part in its inactivation.
c. **True** – by butyrlycholinesterase.
d. **False** – in fact pancuronium inactivates butyrylcholinesterase.
e. **False** – alcuronium undergoes little or no metabolism in the body; it is excreted mainly via the kidneys.

2.70 Answers

a. **True** – an allosteric effect is one that is produced by binding of an agent to a site other than the primary binding site.
b. **True**.
c. **True** – on high doses or where there is decreased breakdown.
d. **True**.
e. **True**.

2.71 Answers

a. **True** – it is 'dibucaine', which is the basis of the dibucaine number as a test for atypical pseudocholinesterase.
b. **True**.
c. **False**.
d. **True** – marked inhibition.
e. **True** – but the inhibition is mild and not sufficient to prolong the action of suxamethonium to any clinically significant degree.

2.72 Answers

a. **False** – it is broken down by acetylcholinesterase to choline and acetic acid. It is the choline that undergoes re-uptake into the nerve terminal, not the acetylcholine.
b. **True** – re-uptake accounts for about 60% of released adrenaline.
c. **True** – it is rapidly taken up the neighbouring glial cells and converted to glutamine and then re-synthesised into glutamate.
d. **True**.
e. **True** – this is the basis of the action of selective serotonin re-uptake inhibitors (SSRIs).

2.73 Answers

a. **True**.
b. **True**.
c. **True**.
d. **False** – pure antagonist.
e. **True**.

2.74 Answers

  a. False.
  b. False.
  c. True – morphine-6-glucuronide is a more potent analgesic than morphine.
  d. True – norpethidine, apart from its muscle rigidity-promoting effect, is also an analgesic.
  e. False – remifentanil's metabolites are, for all practical purposes, inactive.

2.75 Answers

  a. True.
  b. False.
  c. False – it is more common at induction.
  d. False – difficulty of patient ventilation results from hypertonus of pharyngeal and laryngeal muscles than from rigidity of chest wall musculature.
  e. True.

2.76 Answers

  a. True.
  b. False – it increases it.
  c. False – it decreases it.
  d. True.
  e. False.

2.77 Answers

  a. True – propofol is achiral.
  b. True – all the others are cerebral depressants.
  c. True.
  d. False – both methohexitone and thiopentone are anti-analgesics.
  e. True – but this is the effect of the additive propylene glycol rather than the agent itself.

2.78 Answers

  a. True – it has a pH about 10.5.
  b. True – it is about 7.0.
  c. True – keto-enol tautomerism. On injection into the plasma (pH 7.4) thiopentone attracts hydrogen ions and converts to a non-ionised state which isomerises from the keto- form to the enol-form to form a highly lipid soluble compound that easily crosses the blood–brain barrier to exert its anaesthetic effect.
  d. True – see **c**.
  e. True – about 17% on first pass through the lungs.

2.79 Answers

    a. True.
    b. False.
    c. True.
    d. False.
    e. False – propofol is an analgesic (in smaller doses) as much as an anaesthetic.

2.80 Answers

    a. True.
    b. True.
    c. True.
    d. False.
    e. False.

2.81 Answers

    a. True.
    b. True.
    c. False – it is present in thiopentone sodium.
    d. False.
    e. True – it is present along with hydrochloric acid so as adjust the pH.

2.82 Answers

    a. True – in the arterioles of c. 200 μm in diameter.
    b. False – the primary sensor is in the smooth muscle cells, because the phenomenon can occur even in the absence of intact endothelium.
    c. False – voltage-sensitive potassium (K_v) channels are not essential.
    d. False – the hypoic pulmonary vasoconstriction (HPV) response is present in fetal lung and is critical for minimising perfusion of the lung in utero.
    e. False – it is aggravated by ET-1.

2.83 Answers

a. **False** – aspirin does not inactivate lipoxygenase.
b. **True** – aspirin is a non-specific NSAID.
c. **True** – it inactivates cyclo-oxygenase and thereby impairs platelet adhesiveness and thus reduces the efficacy of platelet plugs. It also causes hypoprothrombinaemia by a warfarin-like effect on the vitamin K epoxide cycle.
d. **True** – the respiratory acidosis results from increased metabolism following uncoupling of oxidative phosphorylation. The metabolic acidosis results from increased production of a variety of acids including pyruvic, lactic and phosphoric acids.
e. **True** – aspirin lowers body temperature by its conventional anti-pyretic action. It raises body temperature by increasing metabolism and also, in overdosage, by rendering the thermoregulatory centres ineffective.

2.84 Answers

a. **True** – even several hours after ingestion.
b. **False** – forced diuresis is beneficial in aspirin overdosage, not paracetamol overdosage.
c. **True** – because acute renal failure is a consequence of paracetamol overdosage.
d. **True** – N-acetylcysteine, a sulphur containing amino acid, is a sulphydryl donor and helps 'neutralise' N-acetyl benzquinoneimine, the toxic hepatic metabolite of paracetamol.
e. **True** – because severe liver damage may be associated with bleeding tendency secondary to impaired vitamin K activity.

2.85 Answers

a. **False** – diclofenac does not possess an 'asymmetric' carbon atom.
b. **True** – it is 'dichloro-anilino-phenyl acetic acid'.
c. **True**.
d. **False**.
e. **False** – less than 1% is unchanged diclofenac, the rest is as metabolites.

2.86 Answers

a. **True** – Xenon: 0.14; N_2O: 0.47.
b. **False** – Xenon: 71 %; N_2O: 105%.
c. **True** – because xenon has a greater density: 5.887 g L^{-1}, compared with N_2O: 1.530 g L^{-1}.
d. **True** – Xenon: 1.9; N_2O: 1.4.
e. **False** – Neither agent is known to undergo biotransformation.

2.87 Answers

a. **True** – infant: c. 3.3 ml/kg; adult: 2.0–2.2 ml/kg.
b. **True** – a neonate loses c. 15% of its body water per day, an adult c. 4–5%.
c. **True** – a neonate has about twice the body surface area per unit mass.
d. **True** – neonate: c. 18–20%; adult: c. 9–10%.
e. **True** – neonate: 80–100 ml/kg; adult: c. 70–80 ml/kg.

2.88 Answers

a. **False** – hypocapnia is a more likely pointer to hypotension than hypercapnia.
b. **True** – mental confusion could result from cerebral hypoxia due to poor cerebral perfusion.
c. **True** – because of diminution in coronary blood flow from reduced coronary perfusion pressure.
d. **True** – nausea is sometimes associated with acute hypotension.
e. **False** – respiratory difficulty is not a sign of hypotension per se.

2.89 Answers

a. **False** – movement of the chest is a *necessary* requirement for ventilation but not a *sufficient* requirement. There must also be a patent airway.
b. **False** – the breathing bag can be made to move more or move less by, respectively, decreasing or increasing the fresh gas flow rate for the same respiratory efforts of the patient.
c. **False** – this would only be true if the FiO_2 was the same as that of atmospheric air, i.e. 21%. Most patients under general anaesthesia are likely to have an FiO_2 in the region of 30% or more.
d. **True** – there is no way of maintaining normocapnia other than by adequate ventilation.
e. **False** – peripheral cyanosis may be the result of stagnant hypoxia or red cell polycythaemia.

2.90 Answers

a. **False** – it is the proximal muscles, e.g. the ocular muscles that are chiefly affected.
b. **False** – pain is not a feature of the condition.
c. **False** – it is more likely to be worse in the pre-menstrual phase.
d. **False** – unlike in the Eaton–Lambert (myasthenic) syndrome, muscle wasting is absent.
e. **False**.

Practice paper 3

Anatomy

3.1 The following statements are true:

   a. All the intrinsic muscles of the eye are supplied by the third cranial nerve.
   b. All the intrinsic muscles of the larynx are supplied by the recurrent laryngeal nerve.
   c. The atrioventricular bundle is the sole conductive pathway between the atria and ventricles of the heart.
   d. The sole sensory and motor supply to the diaphragm is by way of the phrenic nerve.
   e. Only one cranial parasympathetic nerve has its origin in the midbrain.

3.2 The following intracranial venous sinuses are paired structures:

   a. Cavernous sinus.
   b. Basilar sinus.
   c. Anterior intercavernous sinus.
   d. Occipital sinus.
   e. Transverse sinus.

3.3 Concerning the arterial blood supply to the spinal cord:

   a. The supply to the cervical part comes via the internal carotid arteries.
   b. The posterior spinal arteries always arise from the vertebral arteries.
   c. The anterior spinal artery supplies predominantly the peripheral part of the cord.
   d. The largest contribution to the anterior spinal artery arises in the cervical region.
   e. Both the ventral and dorsal radicular arteries lie on the anterior aspect of the spinal cord.

3.4 Concerning the cranial parasympathetic outflow:

a. The Edinger–Westphal nucleus is the nerve centre for accommodation for near vision.
b. The superior salivary nucleus has its fibres conveyed in the facial nerve.
c. The inferior salivary nucleus fibres relay in the optic ganglion.
d. The greater petrosal nerve is the nerve of lacrimation.
e. The vagus nerve supplies the large intestine as far down as the sigmoid colon.

3.5 The following nerve tracts contain fibres that cross to the opposite side within the spinal cord:

a. Lateral cortico-spinal tract.
b. Sympathetic pre-ganglionic motor fibres.
c. Spinothalamic tract.
d. Dorsal column-medial lemniscus pathway.
e. Ventral (anterior) cortico-spinal tract.

3.6 The Na^+–K^+–ATPase pump:

a. Is an electrogenic pump.
b. Is a symport system.
c. In most epithelial cells is situated on the luminal edge of the cell.
d. Is an essential prerequisite for glucose absorption in the gut.
e. Owes its activity predominantly to its β subunit.

3.7 NMDA (N-Methyl-D-aspartate) receptors:

a. Are a type of ionotropic receptor.
b. Mediate excitatory transmission.
c. Have high affinity for glutamate.
d. As a rule show high permeability for calcium ions.
e. Are blocked by xenon.

3.8 Glutamate receptors:

a. Have a wide distribution in the CNS.
b. Are all ligand-gated ion channels.
c. Include AMPA receptors.
d. Are excitatory receptors.
e. Are the site of action of ketamine.

3.9 The following are ion channel receptors:

a. Nicotinic acetylcholine receptors.
b. GABA receptors.
c. AMPA receptors.
d. G protein-coupled receptors.
e. Tyrosine kinase receptors.

3.10 In the case of the nicotinic acetylcholine receptor (nAChR):

a. It is a voltage-gated ion channel.
b. It is the receptor present at all autonomic ganglia.
c. It has a heptameric structure.
d. All its subunits are glycosylated.
e. It requires ligand binding to both its α subunits for channel opening to occur.

3.11 cAMP (cyclic adenosine 3′-5′monophosphate):

a. Is an intracellular messenger.
b. Is present in both eukaryotic and prokaryotic cells.
c. Is a structural analogue of parathyroid hormone.
d. Mediates most of its actions through activation of protein kinase.
e. Shows enhanced activity in the presence of methylxanthines.

3.12 The chloride level is higher in the following compared with that of arterial blood plasma:

a. Mixed venous blood.
b. Interstitial fluid.
c. Cerebrospinal fluid.
d. Hepatic cells.
e. Gastric juice in the fasting state.

3.13 Acidification of the urine will enhance the elimination of the following by renal excretion:

a. Aspirin.
b. Amphetamine.
c. Barbiturates.
d. Tricyclic antidepressants.
e. Local anaesthetics.

3.14   Concerning erythropoietin:

   a. It is manufactured by Kupffer cells of the liver.
   b. Its secretion is facilitated by α-adrenergic agonism.
   c. Its secretion is stimulated by androgens.
   d. Its production is inhibited by theophylline.
   e. It is inactivated by the endothelial cells of the renal cortical peritubular capillaries.

3.15   The following increase renin secretion:

   a. Sympathetic stimulation.
   b. Prostaglandins.
   c. A rise in plasma potassium.
   d. Angiotensin II.
   e. Vasopressin.

3.16   Ethanol:

   a. Has a high volume of distribution.
   b. Is subject to zero order kinetics.
   c. Undergoes 100% oxidation in the body.
   d. Potentiates $5HT_3$ receptor activity.
   e. Decreases the plasma concentration of low-density lipoproteins.

3.17   The following drugs enhance the effects of alcohol:

   a. Aspirin.
   b. Cimetidine.
   c. Metoclopramide.
   d. Antihistamines.
   e. Phenothiazines.

3.18   In the case of the heart:

   a. Its predominant autonomic influence is sympathetic.
   b. Its predominant parasympathetic muscarinic receptor subtype is M_2.
   c. Its sympathetic innervation is more prominent in the atria than in the ventricles.
   d. Its sympathetic receptor subtype is solely β_1.
   e. Its autonomic receptors are essentially all G protein-coupled receptors.

3.19 **In the case of action potentials of cardiac tissue:**

a. Slow-response action potentials are confined to the cells of the sinoatrial and atrioventricular nodes.
b. The resting potential is determined by the transmembrane Na^+ gradient.
c. The resting membrane potential is more negative for the special conducting fibres.
d. The plateau phase (Phase 2) results solely from Ca^{2+} influx through L-type calcium channels.
e. Spontaneous depolarisation is a feature only of pacemaker cells.

3.20 **The following are features common to cardiac and skeletal muscle:**

a. Presence of cross-striations.
b. Presence of actin and myosin in their myofibrils.
c. Display a 'plateau phase' in their action potentials.
d. Decreased permeability for K^+ during early phase of action potential.
e. Possession of calcium-sodium channels.

3.21 **In the case of the arterial system:**

a. The mean blood pressure is higher than the arithmetic average of the sum of systolic and diastolic blood pressures.
b. The mean pressure is site dependent.
c. The arterioles account for about 50% of the diastolic pressure.
d. The pulse pressure wave progressively flattens down the arterial tree.
e. The systolic pressure in the ascending aorta is higher than that in the dorsal pedis artery in the recumbent subject.

3.22 **The mean arterial blood pressure:**

a. Is site dependent in the supine subject.
b. Is equal to the diastolic blood pressure + one-third pulse pressure.
c. In a graphic representation of BP is equal to the area under the pressure curve divided by the cardiac period.
d. Decreases with increasing distance from the aortic valve.
e. Is much higher in the aortic arch than in the left ventricle.

3.23 When using a mercury sphygmomanometer a falsely high systolic blood pressure reading is obtained in the following situations:

a. Using a narrow cuff.
b. Applying the cuff loosely round the arm.
c. Applying cuff over several layers of clothing.
d. Deflating the cuff too slowly during measurement.
e. Placing the zero reference point of the sphygmomanometer below heart level.

3.24 Of the three zones of the liver, Zone 3 cells:

a. Have the lowest density of cytochrome P 450 proteins.
b. Are the most susceptible to hypoxia.
c. Are most immune from damage by alcohol.
d. Are the site of 'centrilobular necrosis'.
e. Are most likely to suffer in halothane hepatitis.

3.25 In the case of acetylcholine:

a. It is synthesised intraneuronally from acetyl co-enzyme A.
b. It requires Ca^{2+} as the exocytotic trigger for its release.
c. It requires depolarisation of its pre-synaptic terminal for its release.
d. All of its receptors are ion gated.
e. It undergoes spontaneous in vivo hydrolysis to choline and acetic acid.

3.26 The following are the effects of α_1 agonism:

a. Arteriolar constriction.
b. Uterine contraction.
c. Renin secretion.
d. Hepatic glycogenolysis.
e. Non-shivering thermogenesis.

3.27 The following are effects of β_2 agonism:

a. Skeletal muscle vasodilatation.
b. Bronchodilatation.
c. Lipolysis.
d. Piloerection.
e. Sudomotor activity.

3.28 The following agents produce their effect in part at least by enhancing the actions of adrenaline and noradrenaline:

a. Cocaine.
b. Dopamine.
c. Ephedrine.
d. Metaraminol.
e. Phenylephrine.

3.29 The following are partial agonists:

a. Suxamethonium.
b. Flumazenil.
c. Naloxone.
d. Buprenorphine.
e. Nalbuphine.

3.30 During quiet spontaneous ventilation the following muscles play an active role:

a. Diaphragm.
b. External intercostals.
c. Internal intercostals.
d. Scalenes.
e. Abdominal wall muscles.

3.31 During normal quiet spontaneous ventilation in the standard adult person in the erect position:

a. More than 20% of the chemical energy (derived from ATP) is converted into mechanical energy.
b. Only about 50% of the mechanical energy is used during the inspiratory phase.
c. Most of the utilised energy is lost as heat.
d. The loss of energy as heat occurs only in the expiratory phase.
e. The total energy for the work of each inspiration is about 1 J.

3.32 The Type II cells of the alveolar epithelium:

a. Are essentially 'stem cells'.
b. Produce surfactant.
c. Function as gas exchange membranes.
d. Are susceptible to oxygen toxicity damage.
e. Secrete heparin.

3.33   Surfactant:

a. Is an amphipathic compound.
b. Is a single chemical compound.
c. Consists solely of saturated fatty acid components.
d. Is secreted by 'constitutive exocytosis'.
e. Has an 'innate immunity' function.

3.34   The pulmonary vascular resistance:

a. Is more evenly distributed across the pulmonary vasculature than is the systemic vascular resistance over the systemic vasculature.
b. May be calculated by applying the principles of Ohm's law.
c. May be determined by applying the factors that form the Hagen–Poiseuille equation.
d. Is correctly expressible as dynes per square centimetre.
e. Is increased by acetylcholine.

3.35   The capillary endothelium secretes the following:

a. Nitric oxide.
b. Histamine.
c. Von Willebrand factor.
d. Interleukins.
e. Thrombomodulin.

3.36   The following are 'fundamental units' under the SI Units system:

a. Metre.
b. Kilogram.
c. Kelvin.
d. Candela.
e. Second.

3.37   The following are non-SI units:

a. Millimetre Hg (as a unit of pressure).
b. Angstrom.
c. Becquerel.
d. Bar.
e. Henry.

3.38 The following are dimensionless entities, i.e. they are mere ratios, percentages or fractions and possess no attached units:

 a. Reynolds' number.
 b. Osmotic coefficient.
 c. Dibucaine number.
 d. Bunsen solubility coefficient.
 e. Diffusion coefficient.

3.39 **The following when graphically represented take the form of an accelerating growth exponential curve:**

 a. Variation of blood viscosity with haematocrit.
 b. Change of saturation vapour pressure of a liquid with ambient temperature.
 c. Latent heat of vaporisation of a liquid with temperature.
 d. Flow rate of a fluid under laminar conditions and the fluid pressure gradient.
 e. Solubility of a gas in a solvent and its partial pressure.

3.40 **The following are graded according to French catheter gauge (FCG):**

 a. Stomach tubes.
 b. Chest drain tubes.
 c. Orotracheal tubes.
 d. Nasogastric tubes.
 e. Robertshaw (red rubber) double lumen tubes.

3.41 **The following will increase with a rise in temperature:**

 a. Speed of light in a vacuum.
 b. Viscosity of a liquid.
 c. Osmolarity of a solution.
 d. Latent heat of vaporisation of a liquid.
 e. Electrical resistance of a metal conductor.

3.42 **Boyle's law:**

 a. Is an expression of the Law of Conservation of Mechanical Energy.
 b. Only applies strictly to an ideal gas.
 c. Does not hold if the change is adiabatic.
 d. Can be applied to calculate the amount of gas in an air cylinder.
 e. Can be applied to determine the internal volume of an oxygen cylinder.

3.43 Electrical impedance ought to be high in the following situations:

a. In theatre footwear so as to prevent electrocution by mains electricity.
b. The operating theatre floor so as to prevent buildup of static electricity.
c. In the electrodes used when using a peripheral nerve stimulator to test for neuromuscular blockade.
d. When using ECG electrodes to obtain an ECG display on the monitor.
e. Under a diathermy pad during use of diathermy (electrosurgery).

3.44 The following are features common to the Clark electrode and the fuel cell as methods of oxygen measurement:

a. They both require an 'external' potential difference.
b. They both estimate oxygen in 'partial pressure' units.
c. With oxygen in both devices, the same reaction occurs.
d. They are both temperature sensitive.
e. The measurements in both devices are affected by the presence of inhalational anaesthetic agents.

3.45 The following are physical phenomena relevant to fibreoptic transmission of light:

a. Total internal reflection.
b. Refractive index.
c. Graded indexation of fibres.
d. Coherence.
e. Precession.

3.46 The following are interchangeable on an anaesthetic machine as between the different cylinder gas supplies and their flow paths:

a. Flowmeter tubes.
b. Flow unit bobbins.
c. Bourdon pressure gauges.
d. Bodok seals.
e. Pressure regulators.

3.47 When fitting a fresh oxygen cylinder to an anaesthetic machine:

a. The cylinder needs to be inverted several times before being attached.
b. The cylinder ought to be 'cracked'.
c. After engaging the cylinder to its yoke the cylinder ought to be opened slowly.
d. Overtightening the valve ought to be avoided.
e. The valve ought to be left fully open when the cylinder is ready for use.

3.48 In the case of nitrous oxide cylinders:

    a. They have a pin index head throughout their size range.
    b. They have a filling ratio of about 0.75 in the UK.
    c. Their pressure gauge can give an accurate indication of the cylinder contents.
    d. They can safely be made of aluminium.
    e. They can suffer the Joule–Thomson effect during their use.

3.49 The following gases are produced for medical use by the fractional distillation of air:

    a. Oxygen.
    b. Nitrogen.
    c. Carbon dioxide.
    d. Helium.
    e. Xenon.

3.50 Helium:

    a. In its atomic form is in effect an alpha particle.
    b. When mixed with 21% oxygen in a cylinder ('heliox'), it is in liquid form.
    c. Can be used safely as a peritoneal cavity insufflation gas at laparoscopy providing no diathermy is being used.
    d. Is an integral element in the functioning of the CO_2 laser.
    e. If breathed will cause an alteration in voice pitch.

3.51 Of the medical gases oxygen, nitrogen, helium, carbon dioxide and xenon:

    a. Oxygen is the only one that can behave as a diradical.
    b. Carbon dioxide is the only gas with a critical temperature above 0°C.
    c. Xenon is the only one that has narcotic properties under any pressure.
    d. Helium is the only one that does not solidify, even on cooling to very low temperatures.
    e. Carbon dioxide is the only one that is not obtained by fractional distillation of air.

3.52 The Desflurane 'TEC Mark 6' vaporiser:

    a. Is a 'dual-circuit' vaporiser.
    b. Must necessarily be electrically energised.
    c. Is thermostatically controlled.
    d. Is pressurised at about 2000 cm water pressure.
    e. Is electromechanically coupled between its fresh gas flow rate and desflurane vapour pressure.

3.53 The following contaminants are known to accumulate in low-flow breathing attachments as a result of anaesthetic agent reaction with soda lime:

a. Acetone.
b. Nitrogen dioxide.
c. Bromochlorodifluoroethylene.
d. Carbon monoxide.
e. Water.

3.54 The following are phenomena associated with the different methods of gas monitoring:

a. Pressure broadening.
b. Cross-interference.
c. Precession.
d. Population inversion.
e. Cavitation.

3.55 The following methods of gas analysis can be used to estimate oxygen:

a. Mass spectrometry.
b. Infra-red analysis.
c. Cell polarography.
d. Piezoelectric adsorption.
e. Raman scattering.

3.56 CO_2-induced cerebral vasodilatation:

a. Is mediated by NO of neuronal origin.
b. Is essentially due to pH change.
c. Is dose related in clinical range as manifested by a rise in CBF.
d. Will help reduce ischaemic injury to neurones.
e. Can be attenuated by indomethacin.

3.57 The CMR is suppressed in a dose-related manner by the following anaesthetic agents:

a. Halothane.
b. Thiopentone.
c. Enflurane.
d. Ketamine.
e. Nitrous oxide.

3.58 Arachidonic acid:

   a. Is an unsaturated fatty acid.
   b. Is an eicosanoid.
   c. Is derived from linoleic acid.
   d. Gives rise to leukotrienes.
   e. Is released from neuronal membranes in neuronal ischaemic damage.

3.59 Nitric oxide:

   a. Is a free radical.
   b. Requires NADPH for its production.
   c. Produces its effect by activating adenylate cyclase.
   d. Can positively modulate nociceptor activation.
   e. Is produced by cardiac myocytes.

3.60 The following are examples of competitive antagonism in respect of drug action:

   a. Reversal of non-depolarising NMBAs with neostigmine.
   b. Heparin reversal with protamine sulphate.
   c. Reversal of the effects of histamine with adrenaline.
   d. Reversal of warfarin with vitamin K.
   e. Use of atropine to counteract the bradycardia of β-adrenergic blockers.

3.61 The side effects of warfarin include the following:

   a. Skin necrosis.
   b. Thrombocytopenia.
   c. 'Purple toe' syndrome.
   d. Osteoporosis.
   e. Hyperkalaemia.

3.62 The following have been known to produce desensitisation block at nicotinic acetylcholine receptor sites:

   a. Alcohol.
   b. Anticholinesterases.
   c. Barbiturates.
   d. Local anaesthetics.
   e. Verapamil.

3.63 Suxamethonium:

a. Is a pure competitive antagonist.
b. Owes its rapidity of onset of action essentially to its low lipid solubility.
c. Owes its short duration of action entirely to breakdown by butyrylcholinesterase.
d. Has a shorter duration of action in pregnancy.
e. On enzymatic breakdown produces an active metabolite.

3.64 Vecuronium:

a. Is pancuronium with an added quaternary methyl group.
b. Forms a precipitate when mixed with thiopentone solution.
c. Depends essentially on renal excretion for cessation of activity.
d. On biotransformation produces a metabolite with NM blocking properties.
e. Has been known to cause a polyneuropathy.

3.65 The following are reliable clinical tests of recovery from NM blockade:

a. Ability to protrude tongue.
b. Sustained leg lift for 5 seconds.
c. Ability to maintain a normal tidal volume.
d. Ability to create an inspiratory pressure gradient of 20 cm H_2O.
e. Ability to effect a loud cough.

3.66 The following are essential prerequisites for accurate evaluation of neuromuscular block when using a peripheral nerve stimulator.

a. The stimulus must be supramaximal.
b. Stimulation must be by means of a constant current, not constant voltage.
c. The pulse duration ought to be about 200 ms.
d. The patient must be asleep.
e. The PNS must be battery operated, not mains operated.

3.67 In Train-of-Four (TOF) stimulation:

a. Four successive twitch stimuli are delivered in a total time of 0.5 seconds.
b. The second twitch disappears at about 90% block.
c. Absence of the fourth twitch represents about 50% block.
d. Its sensitivity in visual evaluation of fade is better than that in double-burst stimulation (DBS).
e. Fade following suxamethonium signifies Phase II block.

3.68 Anticholinesterases (given on their own):

a. Can produce a bradycardia.
b. Can induce muscle fasciculations.
c. Can reverse the effects of suxamethonium.
d. Can help reverse some of the effects of poisoning by tricyclic antidepressants.
e. Can produce muscle paralysis in their own right.

3.69 Aspirin inactivates the following enzymes:

a. Cyclo-oxygenase 1 (COX1).
b. Cyclo-oxygenase 2 (COX2).
c. Phospholipase A_2.
d. Lipoxygenase.
e. Thromboxane synthase.

3.70 Leukotrienes:

a. Are unsaturated fatty acids.
b. Are COX dependent for their production.
c. Are reduced in production by a direct action of corticosteroids.
d. Are potent coronary vasodilators.
e. Include the slow-reacting substance of anaphylaxis (SRS-A).

3.71 Of the halogenated inhalational anaesthetics halothane, enflurane, isoflurane, sevoflurane and desflurane:

a. Halothane is the only halogenated alkane.
b. Enflurane is the only one that is reputed to be epileptogenic.
c. Isoflurane is the only one that has ever shown the 'coronary steal syndrome.'
d. Sevoflurane is the only one that is achiral.
e. Desflurane is the least stable with soda lime.

3.72 Halothane:

a. Is a substituted ether.
b. Contains thymol as a preservative.
c. Must be provided in dark bottles to prevent breakdown by light.
d. Is the only inhalational halogenated anaesthetic agent that produces bromochlorodifluoroethylene (BCDFE) with soda lime.
e. Produces 'halothane hepatitis' because of its conversion to trifluoroacetic acid, CF_3COOH.

3.73 The main biotransformation metabolite of the following agents is glucuronide:

a. Thiopentone.
b. Methohexitone.
c. Propofol.
d. Etomidate.
e. Ketamine.

3.74 The following induction agents possess analgesic properties:

a. Thiopentone.
b. Methohexitone.
c. Propofol.
d. Ketamine.
e. Etomidate.

3.75 Each of the following anaesthetic induction agents contains the additive listed against it to render the agent soluble in water:

a. Thiopentone: sodium carbonate.
b. Methohexitone: sodium carbonate.
c. Propofol: soya bean oil.
d. Etomidate: propylene glycol.
e. Ketamine: benzethonium chloride.

3.76 The following are true with regard to thiopentone:

a. It is a malonyl urea compound as well as a piperidine derivative.
b. It displays keto-enol tautomerism.
c. It owes its hypnotic activity to its basic barbiturate ring.
d. It owes its rapidity of onset of action to the presence of sulphur in its structure.
e. It precipitates in vivo because of its extreme alkalinity.

3.77 Thiopentone:

a. On injection undergoes easy dissolution in the plasma.
b. Predominantly affects the rate of respiration rather than its depth.
c. Causes hypotension primarily by diminishing systemic vascular resistance.
d. Acts on voltage-sensitive sodium channels as part of its mode of anaesthetic action.
e. When bound to plasma proteins is mainly bound to globulins.

3.78 The following local anesthetics are chiral compounds:

a. Amethocaine.
b. Bupivacaine.
c. Lidocaine (lignocaine).
d. Prilocaine.
e. Ropivacaine.

3.79 The activity of local anaesthetic agents is generally reduced:

a. In infancy.
b. In pregnancy.
c. In old age.
d. Following myocardial infarction.
e. In malignant disease.

3.80 Tramadol:

a. Is a synthetic analogue of codeine.
b. Has a roughly equal effect at all three types of opioid receptors.
c. Activates spinal inhibition of pain by a mechanism similar to that of tricyclic antidepressants.
d. Causes less respiratory depression than other opioids.
e. Has minimal effects on GI motor function.

3.81 Pruritus associated with opioids:

a. Is μ-receptor mediated.
b. Is necessarily histamine related.
c. May present as facial pruritus, even after spinal opioids.
d. Is reversible with naloxone.
e. Is relieved by ondansetron.

3.82 The respiratory depression caused by the following opioids shows a 'ceiling effect':

a. Buprenorphine.
b. Fentanyl.
c. Morphine.
d. Nalbuphine.
e. Pentazocine.

3.83 The following benzodiazepines produce active metabolites:

a. Diazepam.
b. Midazolam.
c. Lorazepam.
d. Oxazepam.
e. Temazepam.

3.84   Midazolam:

    a. In vivo is less soluble than diazepam.
    b. Is only moderately protein-bound in the plasma.
    c. Displaces diazepam from its receptor site by competitive antagonism.
    d. Is best avoided in porphyria.
    e. On biotransformation produces toxic metabolites.

3.85   Insulin cell-surface receptors are located in the cells of:

    a. Liver.
    b. Skeletal muscle.
    c. Adipose tissue.
    d. Circulating red cells.
    e. Brain.

3.86   In the case of sulphonylurea antidiabetic agents:

    a. Their action is enhanced by alcohol.
    b. Their effects are counteracted by salicylates.
    c. They intensify the action of clofibrate.
    d. They induce a flush following alcohol ingestion.
    e. They induce hyponatraemia.

3.87   The following are true of erythrocytes and their activity:

    a. Their energy substrate under any conditions is solely glucose.
    b. Their metabolic activity can lead only as far as the stage of glycolysis.
    c. Their glucose uptake is insulin dependent.
    d. The movement of HCO_3^- and chloride shifts as part of the Hamburger phenomenon occur via the same ion channel.
    e. The manufacture of haemoglobin inside red cell precursors in the bone marrow occurs entirely inside the cell mitochondria.

3.88   Haemoglobin A1c:

    a. Is merely one of several possible glycated haemoglobin fractions.
    b. Results from enzymatic glucosylation of terminal leucine of the β-globin chain.
    c. Has a half-life of c. 60 days.
    d. Is assayed as grams per decilitre of blood.
    e. Is a more accurate indication of a patient's diabetic status rather than the day-to-day blood sugar level.

3.89 The following are attributes of brown adipose tissue ('brown fat'):

  a. Presence of several small droplets of fat per cell rather than one large fat globule.
  b. Rich sympathetic innervation.
  c. Presence of thermogenin.
  d. Few mitochondria.
  e. Higher level of ATP synthase.

3.90 Hypoxic pulmonary vasoconstriction:

  a. Is a feature only of the human mammal.
  b. Develops only after birth.
  c. Is mediated by mitochondrial electron transport chain in the smooth muscle cells of pulmonary arterioles.
  d. Involves reactive oxygen species as second messengers.
  e. Is relieved by nitric oxide.

3.1 Answers

a. **False** – remember the 'mantra': 'LR 6, SO 4, all the rest by 3': lateral rectus by the sixth (abducens), superior oblique by the fourth (trochlear), all the rest by the third (oculomotor).
b. **False** – the recurrent laryngeal nerve supplies all the laryngeal muscles except the cricothyroid, which is supplied by the external laryngeal branch of the superior laryngeal nerve.
c. **True**.
d. **False** – sole motor supply: phrenic nerve: C3, 4 and 5. The sensory supply to the central part is from the phrenic nerve, and to the periphery is from the lower five intercostal nerves.
e. **True** – the parasympathetic component of the oculomotor nerve originates in the Edinger–Westphal nucleus in the midbrain; the origins of all the others (VII, X and XI) are in the brain stem.

3.2 Answers

a. **True**.
b. **False**.
c. **False**.
d. **True**.
e. **True**.

3.3 Answers

a. **False** – it is via the vertebral arteries.
b. **False** – sometimes they arise from the posterior inferior cerebellar arteries.
c. **False** – it is mainly the central part of the cord.
d. **False** – in the lumbosacral region.
e. **True**.

3.4 Answers

a. **True**.
b. **True**.
c. **True**.
d. **True**.
e. **False** – only as far as the transverse colon.

3.5 Answers

a. **False** – the tract fibres have already crossed in the medulla before descending to the cord.
b. **False** – sympathetic efferent fibres do not cross in the cord.
c. **True**.
d. **False** – the dorsal column tracts cross in the medulla as the medial lemniscus.
e. **True** – this tract does not descend below thoracic level. Most of its fibres cross to the opposite side of the cord before terminating on α and γ motor neurones.

3.6 Answers

a. **True** – because, by extruding 3 Na^+ ions in exchange for 2 K^+ ions, it creates an electrical gradient across the cell membrane.
b. **False** – it is an antiport system because it moves sodium and potassium in opposite directions.
c. **False** – the Na^+–K^+–ATPase pump is situated exclusively on the basolateral membrane of epithelial cells, the only known exception being the choroid plexus where the pump is located on the apical membrane.
d. **True** – the absorption of glucose in the gut (and its re-absorption in the renal tubule) is dependent on the creation of a Na^+ gradient between the gut lumen and the cell, and this is effected by the pump acting at the basolateral membrane.
e. **False** – the α subunit, with a molecular weight of c. 100,000, is the 'active' moiety. It has: (i) three receptor sites on the inside for binding sodium; (ii) two receptor sites on the outside for binding potassium; and (iii) an inside site which has ATPase activity. The function of the β subunit is to anchor the protein complex in the lipid membrane.

3.7 Answers

a. **True**.
b. **True** – in contrast to glycine receptors, which are inhibitory.
c. **True** – in contrast to AMPA receptors, which have low affinity for glutamate.
d. **True** – contrast AMPA receptors, which have low permeability.
e. **True** – xenon, nitrous oxide and ketamine exert their anaesthetic effects by blocking NMDA receptors.

3.8 Answers

a. **True** – they play a major role in excitatory neurotransmission.
b. **False** – ion channels are associated with glutamate receptors and both ligand gating and voltage gating appear to be involved in channel opening.
c. **True** – glutamate receptors are of three types, depending on the agonist: AMPA, NMDA and kainate.
d. **True**.
e. **True** – ketamine binds to its channel and behaves as a non-competitive antagonist.

3.9 Answers

a. **True** – ligand-gated ion channel.
b. **True** – ligand-gated ion channel.
c. **True**.
d. **False**.
e. **False**.

3.10 Answers

a. **False** – it is a ligand-gated ion channel.
b. **True** – it is also found at muscle-cell endplates of the neuromuscular junction and in the CNS.
c. **False** – it is structurally a pentamer, possessing 2 α subunits and one each of β, γ and δ subunits.
d. **True**.
e. **True**.

3.11 Answers

a. **True**.
b. **True**.
c. **False** – it is a structural analogue of thyroid hormone.
d. **True**.
e. **True** – because methylxanthines (e.g. theophylline) inhibit phosphodiesterases, which leads to an increase in cAMP.

3.12 Answers

a. **False** – because of the Hamburger phenomenon: following the conversion of CO_2 to $-HCO_3$ by red cell carbonic anhydrase, bicarbonate moves into the plasma down its concentration gradient and chloride moves into the red cell to maintain electroneutrality (chloride shift). Therefore the venous plasma has a lower chloride content than the arterial plasma.

b. **True** – because of the Gibbs–Donnan effect.

c. **True** – about 15% more than in plasma.

d. **False** – cells generally have less chloride (and bicarbonate) and more phosphate.

e. **True** – the gastric juice chloride is about 155–170 mmol/L.

3.13 Answers

a. **False** – aspirin is better excreted in an alkaline urine.

b. **True**.

c. **False**.

d. **True** – because they are weak bases and therefore more highly ionised in an acid urine.

e. **True** – same as above.

3.14 Answers

a. **True** – and also by hepatocytes, but its main production site is the kidney. See below.

b. **False** – by β-adrenergic agonism.

c. **True**.

d. **True** – adenosine is a stimulant for erythropoietin production. Theophylline is an adenosine antagonist and therefore inhibits erythropoietin production.

e. **False** – the endothelial cells of the peritubular capillaries of the renal cortex are the major site of erythropoietin production.

3.15 Answers

a. **True** – β-adrenergic stimulation.

b. **True** – especially prostacyclin.

c. **False** – the relationship is an inverse one.

d. **False** – reduces its secretion by a negative feedback mechanism.

e. **False** – inhibits its secretion.

3.16 Answers

a. True.
b. True.
c. False – only c. 98%. About 2% of ingested alcohol escapes oxidation and is excreted via the lungs and kidney.
d. True – but only in low concentrations. The action of alcohol is mediated mainly through GABA receptor activity.
e. True – it increases HDLs and lowers LDLs in the plasma.

3.17 Answers

a. False.
b. True – by inhibiting gastric alcohol dehydrogenase.
c. True – by enhancing gastric emptying and thus increasing intestinal absorption of alcohol.
d. True.
e. True.

3.18 Answers

a. False – it is parasympathetic. 'Vagotonia' is the predominant influence on the heart.
b. True.
c. False – more prominent in the ventricles.
d. False – also includes β_2 and β_3.
e. True.

3.19 Answers

a. True.
b. False – by the K^+ gradient.
c. True – c. –90 to –100 mV, compared with –85 to –95 mV for the cardiomyocyte.
d. False – from Ca^{2+} influx as well as K^+ influx through K^+ channels.
e. True.

3.20 Answers

a. True – cross-striations – Z lines – are present in both.
b. True – actin and myosin fibrils in cardiac muscle and skeletal muscle are almost identical and they interdigitate and slide along one another in the same manner in both types of muscle.
c. False – cardiac muscle: yes; skeletal muscle: no.
d. False – cardiac muscle: yes; skeletal muscle: no.
e. False. skeletal muscle does not have calcium-sodium channels.

3.21 Answers

a. **False** – it is lower because diastole is longer than systole.
b. **True** – because both systolic and diastolic pressures vary with the site of measurement.
c. **False** – the arterioles account for about 75–80% of diastolic pressure.
d. **False** – it becomes more peaked.
e. **False** – the systolic pressure in a recumbent subject is slightly higher in the dorsalis pedis artery than in the ascending aorta.

3.22 Answers

a. **True**.
b. **False**.
c. **True**.
d. **True**.
e. **True** – because of the intervention of the aortic valve.

3.23 Answers

a. **True**.
b. **True**.
c. **True**.
d. **False** – it will give a lower than normal reading.
e. **True**.

3.24 Answers

a. **False** – highest density.
b. **True** – because they are furthest away from their source of oxygen viz. hepatic artery and portal vein.
c. **False** – alcohol damage is mediated through hypoxia.
d. **True** – Zone 3 is the centrilobular zone.
e. **True**.

3.25 Answers

a. **True**.
b. **True** – Ca^{2+} is a necessary requirement but not a sufficient requirement. There must also be a Na^+/K^+ exchange at the membrane.
c. **True** – see **b**.
d. **False** – its nicotinic receptor sites are ion gated, while its muscarinic sites are G protein-coupled receptors.
e. **True** – but enzyme (acetyl cholinesterase)-induced breakdown is the normal mode of hydrolysis.

3.26 Answers

a. **True**.
b. **True**.
c. **False** – β_1 agonism.
d. **True**.
e. **False** – Non-shivering thermogenesis, an attribute of brown fat, is the effect of β agonism.

3.27 Answers

a. **True**.
b. **True**.
c. **False** – β_1 effect.
d. **False** – α_1 effect.
e. **False** – α_1 effect, but mediated through acetylcholine.

3.28 Answers

a. **True** – inhibits re-uptake of adrenaline and noradrenaline.
b. **True** – releases noradrenaline at nerve terminals.
c. **True** – on being transported into the pre-synaptic terminal, ephedrine displaces adrenaline, which is then released to bring about its effects.
d. **False** – it is a pure α agonist in its own right.
e. **False** – it is a pure α agonist in its own right.

3.29 Answers

a. **True** – suxamethonium is a partial agonist of the acetylcholine receptor.
b. **False**.
c. **False**.
d. **True** – a partial μ agonist. It antagonises the respiratory depression of fentanyl without completely preventing opioid pain relief.
e. **False** – it is an agonist/antagonist opioid because it is a μ receptor antagonist but a κ_1 and κ_3 agonist (analgesic effect).

3.30 Answers

a. **True**.
b. **True**.
c. **True**.
d. **True** – contrary to previous belief, the scalenes are not accessory muscles of respiration; they are active in inspiration during quiet breathing.
e. **False**.

3.31 Answers

a. **False** – only about 10%.
b. **True** – the rest is stored in the chest and alveolar walls as potential energy, which then provides the 'elastic recoil' for the process of expiration.
c. **True** – c. 90%.
d. **False** – about equally divided between the two phases of ventilation.
e. **True**.

3.32 Answers

a. **True** – they give rise to Type I cells.
b. **True**.
c. **False** – no. They are rounded in shape and are situated at the junction of alveolar septa.
d. **False** – resistant to oxygen toxicity damage.
e. **False** – heparin is produced by mast cells that are situated in the periphery of the capillary endothelium.

3.33 Answers

a. **True** – an amphipathic compound is one that has both hydrophilic and lipophilic moieties.
b. **False** – the primary agent in surfactant is dipalmitoyl phosphatidylcholine; the other agents include fatty acids and proteins.
c. **False** – see **b**.
d. **True** – exocytosis is the process by which secretory granules release their contents at the cell surface by fusing their edges with the surface of the cell. The process may be 'regulated', when the stored granules are released as required in response to a requisite stimulus (secretory granules of acinar cells of pancreas) or 'constitutive', when they are released continuously, as in the case of surfactant.
e. **True**.

3.34 Answers

a. **True** – the SVR resides predominantly (c. 75–80%) in the arterioles. As an approximation, the PVR resides about equally in the arterioles, capillaries and veins.
b. **True** – but only as a rough approximation: Ohm's law: $V = i \times R$. The vascular equivalent of this is: $BP = CO \times SVR$.
c. **True** – yes, as a rough approximation. Again, note that the Hagen–Poiseuille equation: $Q = \pi r^4 P / 8\acute{\eta} L$ is the same as $BP = CO \times SVR$, though arranged differently.
d. **False** – dyne seconds per centimetre^{-5}.
e. **False** – decreased. Acetylcholine is a vasodilator.

3.35 Answers

a. **True**.
b. **True**.
c. **True**.
d. **True**.
e. **True**.

3.36 Answers

a. **True**.
b. **True**.
c. **False**.
d. **False**.
e. **True**.

Note: the reference is to 'fundamental' units, not 'base' units. There are three fundamental quantities of measurement: length, mass and time, and their respective units are: metre, kilogram and second. The whole of mechanics can be expressed in these three units, which are also called 'dimensional' units because length, mass and time are referred to as 'dimensions'.

3.37 Answers

a. **True**.
b. **True** – the angstrom = 0.1 nm.
c. **False** – it is the SI unit of radiation activity of a radionuclide decaying at a rate, on average, of one spontaneous nuclear transition per second.
d. **True**.
e. **False** – the henry is the SI unit of inductance, i.e. the inductance equal to that of a closed circuit in which an electro-motive force (EMF) of 1 V is produced when the current in the circuit varies uniformly at a rate of one ampere per second.

3.38 Answers

a. **True** – Re = $v\rho l / \eta$, where v is the velocity of flow, ρ is the density of fluid, l is the length of tube, and η is the viscosity of fluid.

b. **True** – the osmotic coefficient of a solute is an expression of the degree to which the solute is ionised in solution and therefore influences the osmolality of the solution. Where there is 100% ionisation, the osmotic coefficient is equal to 1; where the ionisation is less than 100% the coefficient is less than 1.

c. **True** – the percentage inhibition of butrylcholinesterase by dibucaine. Normal butryl cholinesterase (BCE): 80%; atypical BCE: 20%.

d. **False** – Bunsen solubility coefficient: volume of gas, corrected to standard temperature and pressure (STP), which dissolves in one unit volume of a liquid at the temperature concerned when the partial pressure of the gas above the liquid is one atmosphere.

e. **False** – the diffusion coefficient of a membrane is the permeability of the membrane (to a particular solute) multiplied by the total area of the membrane.

3.39 Answers

a. **True**.

b. **True**.

c. **False** – the latent heat of vaporisation of a liquid falls with temperature.

d. **False** – the relationship is linear. It is under conditions of turbulent flow that the relationship takes the form of an accelerating positive exponential.

e. **False** – the relationship is a direct linear one.

3.40 Answers

a. **True**.

b. **True**.

c. **False** – according to internal and external diameters in millimetres.

d. **True**.

e. **False** – as small, medium and large. Carlens tubes are graded according to FCG: sizes 35, 37, 39 and 41.

Note: FCG is a unit with dimensions. It is the external circumference of the device in millimetres. SWG has no dimensions; it refers to the number of the particular device that can be accommodated in a standard measuring device. For this reason the higher the SWG number the smaller the bore of the device, e.g. cannulae.

3.41 Answers

a. **False** – the speed of light in a vacuum is unaffected by temperature.
b. **False** – it decreases.
c. **False** – osmolarity is defined with respect to *volume* of solvent. A rise in temperature of a solution will increase its volume and therefore lead to a decrease in osmolarity.
d. **False** – falls with a rise in temperature.
e. **True** – conductors increase their resistance with a rise in temperature.

3.42 Answers

a. **True** – According to Boyle's law $P \times V$ is a constant. $P \times V$ is energy. If the pressure doubles, the volume is halved, so the product remains the same.
b. **True**.
c. **True** – for Boyle's law to hold the temperature of the gas must remain constant. In adiabatic change, there is no movement of heat between the contained gas and the surroundings, therefore there is a rise or fall of temperature depending on whether the gas is being compressed (pressure increases) or is being decompressed (pressure decreases).
d. **False** – this requires application of the Ideal Gas equation: $PV = nRT$.
e. **True** – e.g. a full 137 bar size E oxygen cylinder gives 680 L of oxygen at 1 bar. Therefore it holds a total of $(680 + \alpha)$ L of oxygen, α being the number of litres of oxygen that remain in the cylinder when it is 'empty'. Therefore $137 \times \alpha$ (i.e. the internal volume of the cylinder in litres) = 1 bar $\times$ $(680 + \alpha)$. Therefore $680 + \alpha = 137\alpha$. Therefore $\alpha = 5$ L.

3.43 Answers

a. **True**.
b. **False**.
c. **False** – high impedance will reduce the current.
d. **False**.
e. **False** – high impedance will lead to a high 'current density' and thereby give the patient an electrical diathermy burn.

3.44 Answers

a. **False** – the Clark cell is an 'electrolytic' cell and therefore needs an external electrical source. The fuel cell is a 'voltaic' cell and in effect creates its own potential difference.
b. **True**.
c. **True**.
d. **True**.
e. **True** – halothane in the case of the Clark electrode, N_2O in the case of the fuel cell.

3.45 Answers

a. **True** – it describes the manner in which the light beam is transmitted along the cable.

b. **True** – the refractive index of the light transmitting cable must be higher than that of the cladding enveloping it.

c. **True** – this refers to the gradual 'gradation' of the refractive index of the light-transmitting fibres in their disposition in relation to the centre of the transmitting cable.

d. **True** – if the fibrelight is to transmit a picture, as opposed to providing light for mere illumination, then the fibres must have a fixed and regular relationship to each other right along the length of the cable. This is 'coherence'.

e. **False** – precession is a property of MRI.

3.46 Answers

a. **False** – because the viscosity, density and required flow rate are different for each gas.

b. **False** – as **a**. above.

c. **False** – because the pressures of full cylinders are different for the different gases.

d. **True**.

e. **False** – because the 'upstream' pressures are different for the different gases, although the downstream pressures are the same viz. 400 kPa.

3.47 Answers

a. **False** – this is not necessary for oxygen, but is necessary for entonox cylinders.

b. **True** – 'cracking' is the opening of a cylinder valve very slightly so as to let some of the gas out to blow out any dust in the pin index holes.

c. **True** – this is to prevent adiabatic compression and thus a rise in temperature at the Bodok seal interface.

d. **True** – because it damages the cylinder threads.

e. **True**.

3.48 Answers

a. **False** – only for cylinder sizes C, D and E. F and G have 'cartwheel' heads.

b. **False** – the filling ratio for the UK is 0.65. For the tropics it is 0.75.

c. **False** – because the agent in the cylinder is a mixture of a liquid and a gas.

d. **True** – this is necessary for use in a MRI scanner room.

e. **True**.

3.49 Answers

a. **True**.
b. **True**.
c. **False** – CO_2 is manufactured in the UK: (i) as a by-product gas from manufacture of hydrogen; (ii) as a by-product gas from fermentation; and (iii) as a combustion gas from burning fuel.
d. **False** – essentially from natural gas.
e. **True**.

3.50 Answers

a. **True** – alpha particles are positively charged helium nuclei, i.e. they contain two protons and two neutrons, so they have a charge of +2.
b. **False**.
c. **False** – although helium is non-toxic to the body it is a very insoluble gas and therefore ought not be used for laparoscopic insufflation. The two requirements of such a gas are: (i) it must be non-toxic; and (ii) it must be highly soluble in blood.
d. **True** – it helps maintain 'population inversion', i.e. a higher percentage (population) of energised CO_2 molecules compared with unenergised molecules.
e. **True** – causes a high-pitched voice because of its lower density compared with air.

3.51 Answers

a. **True** – a diradical is a substance that contains two unpaired electrons.
b. **False** – critical temperature of CO_2: 31°C; of xenon: 16.5°C.
c. **False** – at a pressure of 30 atmospheres, nitrogen is narcotic.
d. **True** – that is why helium can be used as the coolant in the MRI scanner.
e. **False** – helium is obtained not from fractional distillation of air, but from natural gas.

3.52 Answers

a. **True** – it has a separate circuit for the fresh gases and anaesthetic vapour.
b. **True** – to heat the liquid agent and to operate the vaporiser controls.
c. **True** – the vapour chamber is maintained at 39°C.
d. **True** – 200 kPa, which is the same as 2000 cm H_2O pressure.
e. **True**.

3.53 Answers

a. **False** – acetone can accumulate but because it is released by the patient.
b. **False** – there may be minute amounts of NO_2 in the cylinder (fresh) gases, but it is not produced by agent reaction with soda lime.
c. **True** – a reaction between halothane and soda lime.
d. **True** – a reaction between desflurane, enflurane, isoflurane and to a lesser extent with sevoflurane with soda lime.
e. **True** – water is a by-product of the reaction of CO_2 with soda lime.

3.54 Answers

a. **True** – it is observed with infra-red gas analysis. Changes in the total pressure of the gas mixture will affect the width of the infra-red absorption bands of individual gases.
b. **True** – this occurs in gas analysis by mass spectrometry. Where similar gases are present there may be overlap of the beams of deflection of different agents.
c. **False** – precession ('wobbling') is a phenomenon of protons during MRI scanning.
d. **False** – population inversion is a laser phenomenon.
e. **False** – during ultrasound imaging high-peak pressures of the US beam can cause microbubbles in tissue liquid to expand to the point of sudden collapse accompanied by high temperatures, resulting in tissue damage: cavitation.

3.55 Answers

a. **True** – mass spectrometry can be used to monitor any gas.
b. **False** – infra-red analysis is only applicable for gases that have two or more dissimilar elements.
c. **True**.
d. **False**.
e. **True** – Raman scattering can be used to monitor any gas that has two or more atoms per molecule.

3.56 Answers

a. **True** – but not exclusively by NO.
b. **True**.
c. **True** – varies directly by 1–2 ml/100 g/minute for each 1 mmHg change in pCO_2.
d. **False** – will worsen it because of loss of the cerebral 'steal' phenomenon.
e. **True** – because the vasodilator response is mediated in part by prostaglandins, and indomethacin blocks prostaglandin activity and can thus reduce the vasodilator response.

3.57 Answers

a. **True**.
b. **True**.
c. **True**.
d. **False**.
e. **False**.

3.58 Answers

a. **True** – it has four carbon–carbon double bonds.
b. **True** – has 20 carbon atoms (*eicosi* in Greek means twenty).
c. **True**.
d. **True** – through the action of lipoxygenase.
e. **True**.

3.59 Answers

a. **True**.
b. **True**.
c. **False** – by activating guanylate cyclase.
d. **True**.
e. **True**.

3.60 Answers

a. **True**.
b. **False**.
c. **False**.
d. **True**.
e. **False**.

Note: drug antagonism may be:

1. Pharmacological: here the antagonist prevents an agonist from interacting with its receptors to produce an effect. The type of antagonism can be *competitive* or *non- competitive*. Competitive antagonists compete with agonists in a reversible fashion for the same receptor site, e.g. **a**. Non-competitive antagonists bind irreversibly to the receptor site or another site so as to inhibit the response to the agonist. No matter how much agonist is given, the action of the antagonist cannot be overcome.

2. Physiological: here the antagonism is to the physiological effect of the agonist and is brought about by the antagonist acting at a *different* receptor, e.g. the reversal of the hypotensive effect of a spinal or epidural (resulting from blockade at the sympathetic ganglia) by the administration of vasoconstrictor e.g. metaraminol, which acts on the peripheral vasomotor receptor sites.

3. Chemical: (also called antagonism by neutralisation). This occurs when the 'agonist' and 'antagonist' combine chemically to form a neutral compound, e.g. (i) heparin reversal by protamine, and **b**., (ii) gastric acid neutralisation by oral citrate.

3.61 Answers

a. **True** – painful erythematous patches on skin, especially in females.
b. **False** – warfarin has no effect on the platelet count. Thrombocytopenia is a side effect of heparin.
c. **True** – results from embolisation of cholesterol from atheromatous plaques, following bleeding into plaques.
d. **False** – it is a side effect of heparin.
e. **False** – it is a side effect of heparin.

3.62 Answers

a. **True**.
b. **True** – in high dosage they can cause high levels of acetylcholine, which is the cause of the block.
c. **True**.
d. **True** – especially cocaine.
e. **True** – presumably by blocking Ca^{2+} channels and thereby diminishing the rate of acetylcholine release.

3.63 Answers

a. **False** – suxamethonium is a partial agonist.
b. **True**.
c. **False** – also to diffusion of the agent away from the site of action.
d. **False** – it has a longer duration of action because of lower levels of butyrylcholinesterase in pregnancy.
e. **True** – succinyl monocholine also has some neuromuscular blocking action.

3.64 Answers

a. **False** – it has one less methyl group than pancuronium.
b. **True**.
c. **False** – only c.15–25% is excreted via the kidneys. The rest undergoes biliary excretion.
d. **True** – the 3-hydroxy metabolite has some neuromuscular blocking activity.
e. **True** – following long-term use in ITU patients.

3.65 Answers

a. **False**.
b. **True**.
c. **False**.
d. **False** – must be about 40 cm H_2O.
e. **True**.

3.66 Answers

a. **True**.
b. **False** – it is preferable but not essential.
c. **False** – about 200 μs. Longer currents can lead to direct stimulation of the muscle.
d. **False** – preferable because the patient will then not feel pain, but it is not essential.
e. **False** – preferable but not essential.

3.67 Answers

a. **False** – the total time of delivery of four successive stimuli is 2.0 seconds.
b. **True**.
c. **False** – it is about 75% block.
d. **False** – sensitivity of evaluation of visual fade in DBS is better than in TOF stimulation.
e. **True**.

3.68 Answers

a. **True** – the bradycardia is profound and can lead to cardiac arrest.
b. **True**.
c. **True** – in Phase II block of suxamethonium.
d. **True**.
e. **True**.

3.69 Answers

a. **True**.
b. **True**.
c. **False**.
d. **False**.
e. **False**.

3.70 Answers

a. **True** – as the name suggests, leukotrienes have three double bonds and were first isolated from white cells.
b. **False** – they are lipoxygenase dependent for their production.
c. **False** – glucocorticoids directly inhibit cyclo-oxygenase, but only indirectly inhibit lipoxygenase, the leukotriene-generating enzyme. This is by an indirect effect, i.e. by inactivating phospholipase A_2, the convertor of phospholipids to arachidonate, an earlier step in the generation of prostanoids and leukotrienes.
d. **False** – leukotrienes cause coronary vasoconstriction and nanomolar concentrations are sufficient for this purpose.
e. **True** – it is LTC_4 and LTD_4.

3.71 Answers

a. True – the others are all halogenated ethers.
b. True.
c. False – enflurane has also been suspected of the 'coronary steal syndrome.'
d. True.
e. True – because desflurane is the agent that produces the most amount of CO with soda lime.

3.72 Answers

a. False – it is a substituted alkane.
b. True.
c. True – it is broken down by UV light.
d. True.
e. True – trifluoroacetic acid, in the form of trifluoroacetylchloride, is a reactive metabolite of halothane, which when coupled to a liver macromolecule forms an immunogen, which causes halothane hepatitis.

3.73 Answers

a. True – it is biotransformed by oxidation, N-dealkylation, desulphuration and destruction of the barbiturate ring. It is then converted in part to glucuronic acid conjugates.
b. True – same as **a**.
c. True – to glucuronide (and sulphate).
d. False – it is metabolised mainly in the liver by esterification to the carboxylate of etomidate and to a lesser degree by D-alkylation.
e. True – it undergoes N-demethylation to norketamine, which is then converted to hydroxyketamine and eventually to the glucuronide.

3.74 Answers

a. False – the agent is in fact an anti-analgesic.
b. False – same as for thiopentone (see **a**).
c. True.
d. True – it is an excellent analgesic.
e. False – etomidate has no analgesic activity.

3.75 Answers

a. **False** – thiopentone is soluble in water. The sodium carbonate does make it more soluble but it is not added for that purpose. Its essential role is to prevent formation of free acid on exposure to air.

b. **False** – same as for thiopentone, see **a**.

c. **False** – propofol is emulsified, not solubilised, by the addition of soya bean oil.

d. **False** – etomidate is soluble in water. The propylene glycol makes the agent more stable.

e. **False** – ketamine is water soluble; the benzethonium chloride is a preservative.

3.76 Answers

a. **True**.

b. **True** – the tautomeric change is essential to render the agent soluble in vivo.

c. **False** – its hypnotic activity is owed to its alkyl side chains.

d. **True**.

e. **True**.

3.77 Answers

a. **False**.

b. **False** – the depth is affected more than the rate. cx. opioids.

c. **False** – primarily by cardiac depression.

d. **True**.

e. **False** – it is mainly bound to albumin.

3.78 Answers

a. **False**.

b. **True**.

c. **False**.

d. **True**.

e. **True**.

3.79 Answers

a. **True**.

b. **True**.

c. **True**.

d. **True**.

e. **True**.

In all of the above conditions there is an increase in plasma α_1-acid glycoprotein, which leads to increased binding of the LA and therefore lower availability of the active form.

3.80 Answers

a. **True** – it is a 4-phenyl-piperidine analogous of codeine.
b. **False** – it stimulates all three types but δ and κ receptors to a lesser extent.
c. **True** – by decreasing re-uptake of noradrenaline and serotonin.
d. **True**.
e. **True**.

3.81 Answers

a. **True**.
b. **False** – (i) non-histamine-releasing opioids also cause pruritus; and (ii) it is also seen after administration of fentanyl, which does not release histamine.
c. **True**.
d. **True**.
e. **True** – it has been known to be ameliorated after administration of ondansetron.

3.82 Answers

a. **True**.
b. **False**.
c. **False**.
d. **True**.
e. **True**.

3.83 Answers

a. **True** – desmethyldiazepam (nordiazepam), temazepam and oxazepam.
b. **True** – hydroxymidazolams.
c. **False** – it produces an inactive 3-O-phenolic glucuronide.
d. **False** – oxazepam produces an inactive glucuronide conjugate.
e. **True** – temazepam is converted to oxazepam by demethylation.

3.84 Answers

a. **False** – midazolam is the only commonly used benzodiazepine that is water soluble.
b. **False** – it is c. 96% protein-bound.
c. **True** – because it has about twice the affinity for benzodiazepine receptors compared with diazepam.
d. **True** – because of doubts about its safety.
e. **False**.

3.85 Answers

a. **True** – c. 300,000 per cell.
b. **True**.
c. **True** – up to c. 300,000 per cell.
d. **True** – c. 40 per red cell.
e. **True** – but the brain does not depend on insulin as a facilitator of glucose ingress into cells, hence the low number of insulin receptors.

3.86 Answers

a. **True** – alcohol causes hypoglycaemia in its own right.
b. **False** – their action is aggravated by salicylates by displacing sulphonylureas from their binding plasma proteins.
c. **True** – by the same mechanism as in **b** above.
d. **True**.
e. **True** – by increasing ADH activity in the renal collecting tubules.

3.87 Answers

a. **True** – the red cells are the only 'organ' in the body that is solely dependent on glucose as their energy substrate at all times.
b. **True** – in the absence of mitochondria the breakdown of glucose cannot proceed beyond glycolysis, because the Krebs cycle can only function in the mitochondria.
c. **False** – red cells, brain cells and liver cells do not depend on insulin for the entry of glucose.
d. **True** – it is a form of facilitated diffusion and is a counter transport system.
e. **False** – in the bone marrow red cell precursor – which has mitochondria that the mature red cell does not have – the first step in the manufacture of haemoglobin is the formation of d aminolaevulinic acid (ALA). This occurs in the mitochondria, after which the ALA moves out into the cytoplasm for the next few steps, and then returns into the mitochondria for the final three steps.

3.88 Answers

a. **True** – there are two further minor glycation fractions, haemoglobin A1a and A1b, and they are assayed by methods different to that for Hb A1c.
b. **False** – results from non-enzymatic glucosylation of terminal valine of the β chain.
c. **True** – because the lifespan of a red cell is about 120 days.
d. **False** – it is assayed as a percentage; the normal value is c. 6%.
e. **True** – glycation of haemoglobin is an irreversible process and therefore the glycated Hb fraction gives an integrated picture of the mean blood glucose level during half the life span of the red cell, i.e. c. 60 days.

3.89 Answers

a. **True** – a single large fat globule per cell is a feature of 'white' fat.
b. **True** – β-adrenergic innervation.
c. **True** – this is a special protein that allows the protons to flow out easily as heat.
d. **False** – it is rich in mitochondria.
e. **False** – it has a lower level of ATP synthase.

3.90 Answers

a. **False** – it is a feature of all mammalian species.
b. **False** – is present in the fetus and is essential to minimise perfusion of the (unventilated) fetal lung.
c. **True**.
d. **True** – probably H_2O_2.
e. **True**.

Practice paper 4

Anatomy

4.1 **The manubrosternal junction (Angle of Louis) is the surface landmark for the following:**

a. High point of the arch of the aorta.
b. Anterior end of the horizontal fissure of the right lung.
c. Origin of the innominate artery.
d. Hooking of right recurrent laryngeal nerve round the subclavian artery.
e. Stellate ganglion.

4.2 **The following are present as distinctive features of the blood–brain barrier:**

a. Fenestrated capillaries.
b. Tight junctions between endothelial cells.
c. Abundant pinocytic vesicles.
d. Intracellular nucleotidases.
e. Glial cells.

4.3 **In the case of the nervous system:**

a. Type A nerve fibres are the typical myelinated fibres of spinal nerves.
b. Type C nerve fibres constitute more than half the sensory fibres in peripheral nerves.
c. Postganglionic autonomic nerves are Type A α;
d. All sensory transmitter nerves cross at spinal cord level before transmission to the brain.
e. The anterolateral and the dorsal sensory system pathways each has the ability to transmit a broad spectrum of sensory modalities.

4.4 **In the case of the eye:**

a. The extrinsic muscles are all supplied by the 4th cranial nerve.
b. The parasympathetic supply arises in the Edinger–Westphal nucleus.
c. The spinal origin of its sympathetic supply is in the intermediolateral horn of the 2nd and 3rd thoracic segments.
d. The elevator superior palpebrae muscle has a dual motor supply.
e. Accommodation results from activity of the ciliary muscle.

4.5   Concerning the foramina of the diaphragm:

a. The aortic opening is more anterior than the oesophageal opening.
b. The oesophageal opening also conveys the vagus nerves.
c. The caval opening is the highest of all.
d. The thoracic duct is contained in the aortic opening.
e. The superior epigastric vessels are transmitted from the thorax to abdomen in the sternocostal gap.

Cardiovascular system

4.6   The mean arterial blood pressure in the recumbent subject:

   a. Can be correctly taken as being equal to the systolic pressure plus one-third the diastolic pressure.
   b. Is higher in the dorsalis pedis artery than in the aorta.
   c. Is lower in the aorta than in the left ventricle.
   d. Is related to the systole–diastole time ratio.
   e. Other things being equal, will be higher with a higher heart rate.

4.7   Concerning the generation sites of the cardiac action potential:

   a. The sinoatrial node has the least negative resting action potential.
   b. The fastest impulse conduction occurs in the Purkinje system.
   c. The phase of spontaneous repolarisation is most prominent in the left ventricular musculature.
   d. The atrial musculature has no time-dependent currents in phase 4.
   e. Retrograde conduction is normally possible in all parts of the conducting system.

4.8   In the case of the systemic circulation:

   a. Its maximal cross-sectional area is at the arteriolar end of the capillaries.
   b. More than 50% of its blood volume is in the veins.
   c. Its steepest pressure drop is across the capillaries.
   d. The aggregate resistance contributed by vessels of a particular order of arborisation depends solely on their average diameter.
   e. Its fenestrae are wider at the arterial end of capillaries than at their venular end.

4.9   The pulmonary capillaries:

   a. Are about 7–8 nm in thickness.
   b. Normally hold about half the blood volume in the pulmonary circulation.
   c. Produce plasminogen activator.
   d. Inactivate both adrenaline and noradrenaline.
   e. Pre-form and store eicosanoids.

4.10 The following are functions performed by the pulmonary capillary endothelium:

a. Phase II biotransformation.
b. Conversion of angiotensinogen into angiotensin I.
c. Inactivation of 5-hydroxytryptamine.
d. Production of nitric oxide.
e. Synthesis of arachidonic acid.

4.11 Compared with 'white' fat, brown fat:

a. Is more abundant in adults than in infants.
b. Contains multiple fat droplets, as opposed to a single large droplet in white fat.
c. Has a rich sympathetic innervation.
d. Has more mitochondria.
e. Contains an additional proton conductance.

4.12 Autonomic α_2 agonism results in:

a. Skeletal muscle vasodilatation.
b. Relaxation of the gut.
c. Increased release of insulin by the pancreas.
d. Increased sweating.
e. Arteriolar constriction.

4.13 The atrioventricular node:

a. Is situated in the right atrium just posterior to the ostium of the coronary sinus.
b. Normally is under greater sympathetic influence than parasympathetic influence.
c. Is well endowed with gap junctions.
d. Has a faster rate of spontaneous depolarisation than the sinoatrial node.
e. Delays impulse conduction because of dependence on slow calcium channels for propagation of its action potential.

4.14 Myoglobin:

a. Has a sigmoid oxygen dissociation curve.
b. Binds one oxygen molecule per myoglobin molecule.
c. Has a lower P_{50} than haemoglobin.
d. Is found in highest concentration in muscles specialised for sustained contraction.
e. Facilitates oxygen diffusion from blood to mitochondria.

4.15 Concerning the carriage of CO_2 in the blood:

    a. Arterial blood has higher volumes per cent of CO_2 than of oxygen.

    b. CO_2 combining with haemoglobin to form carbaminohaemoglobin is enzyme dependent.

    c. CO_2 conversion to $-HCO_3$ is essentially a reaction in the plasma.

    d. The amount carried as carbonic acid per se is extremely small.

    e. The highest percentage of CO_2 carriage is in the form of carbaminohaemoglobin.

4.16 Concerning albumin:

    a. Over 50% of the albumin pool is in the plasma compartment.

    b. It contains disulphide bonds in its structure.

    c. It is an oxygen free-radical scavenger.

    d. It is essential for maintaining normal capillary permeability.

    e. It binds acidic drugs.

4.17 The following are inactivated during passage through the pulmonary circulation:

    a. Adenosine.

    b. Adrenaline.

    c. Angiotensin II.

    d. Atrial natriuretic peptide.

    e. Noradrenaline.

4.18 The following increase vasopressin release by the posterior pituitary:

    a. Hypovolaemia.

    b. Hypernatraemia

    c. Morphine.

    d. Alcohol.

    e. Angiotensin II.

4.19 The carotid body:

    a. Has the highest blood flow in relation to mass of any organ.

    b. Has Hering's nerve as its afferent pathway.

    c. Can act as a baroreceptor as well.

    d. Is a more powerful chemo-sensor than the central respiratory chemoreceptors.

    e. Is faster in its response to blood gas changes than are the central chemoreceptors.

4.20 Cerebral ischaemia leads to the following changes inside neurones:

a. Rise in intraneuronal calcium.
b. Release of arachidonic acid.
c. Release of nitric oxide.
d. Oxidative injury to DNA.
e. Lactic acidosis.

4.21 The capillary endothelium in the following organs is fenestrated:

a. Heart.
b. Lungs.
c. Liver.
d. Brain.
e. GI tract.

4.22 In the case of the liver:

a. Zone 1 (the periportal zone) is the chief site of ammonia production.
b. Biotransformation of xenobiotics takes place mainly in Zone 3.
c. Zone 2 hepatocytes have the highest content of CYP 450.
d. Hypoxia is more likely to give rise to necrosis of Zone 3 cells.
e. Zone 2 necrosis gives rise to the highest fall in GST levels.

4.23 The liver is responsible for synthesis of the following factors involved in blood coagulation:

a. Factor III.
b. Factor IV.
c. Von Willebrand factor.
d. Protein C.
e. Protein S.

4.24 The intestinal absorption of glucose:

a. Is insulin dependent.
b. Resembles the process of re-absorption in the renal proximal tubule.
c. Requires phosphorylation.
d. Is markedly dependent on concomitant sodium absorption.
e. Is essentially normal in diabetes mellitus.

4.25 Consumption of alcohol leads to the following:

a. A metabolic acidosis.
b. Increase in hepatic gluconeogenesis.
c. Decrease in activity of the Krebs' citric acid cycle.
d. Increased oxidation of fatty acids.
e. Increase in renal uric acid excretion.

4.26 During starvation the following can and do utilise ketone bodies as their energy substrate:

a. Brain cells.
b. Cardiac myocytes.
c. Liver cells.
d. Kidney cells.
e. Red cells.

4.27 The Na^+–K^+–ATPase pump is an essential prerequisite for the following:

a. Maintenance of the integrity of the intracellular fluid compartment (ICF) volume.
b. Absorption of glucose in the gut lumen.
c. Re-absorption of amino acids in the renal tubule.
d. Positive inotropic effect of digoxin.
e. Secretion of hydrochloric acid in the stomach.

4.28 During normal quiet spontaneous ventilation in the standard adult subject in the erect position:

a. The diaphragm is the only active muscle during inspiration.
b. The intrapleural pressure remains subatmospheric in both phases of ventilation.
c. The anatomical and physiological dead space volumes are about equal.
d. Expended energy is lost as heat only in the inspiratory phase.
e. Expiration is a passive process.

4.29 Type I alveolar cells:

a. Give rise to Type II cells.
b. Are oxygen susceptible.
c. Produce surfactant.
d. Produce heparin.
e. Produce ACE for converting angiotensin I to angiotensin II.

4.30 **Static compliance with respect to respiration:**

    a. Is the reciprocal of resistance.
    b. Is the change in lung volume divided by the peak airway pressure.
    c. Can be measured by simple spirometry and manometry.
    d. 'Total compliance' is the sum of lung compliance and chest wall compliance.
    e. Is increased with prolonged breathing of high oxygen concentrates.

4.31 **Angiotensin II:**

    a. Is a decapeptide.
    b. Has a half-life of about 20–30 minutes in the plasma.
    c. Is a more potent vasoconstrictor than adrenaline.
    d. Penetrates the blood–brain barrier.
    e. Facilitates noradrenaline release from postganglionic sympathetic nerve endings.

4.32 **Erythropoietin:**

    a. Is a pure polypeptide.
    b. Is produced solely in the kidney.
    c. Has a circulation half-life of about 20 minutes.
    d. Is facilitated in its secretion by β-adrenergic stimulation.
    e. Is inactivated mainly in the liver.

4.33 **Nitric oxide:**

    a. Is an amphiphilic substance.
    b. Is synthesised in the brain.
    c. Is a powerful vasorelaxant.
    d. Has potent anti-platelet action.
    e. Is capable of both autocrine and paracrine effects.

4.34 **Eicosanoids:**

    a. Are 20-carbon fatty acids.
    b. In the main are saturated fatty acids.
    c. Are normally present in the body in their *trans* isomeric form.
    d. Include the thromboxanes.
    e. Exclude SRS-A (the slow-reacting substance of anaphylaxis).

4.35 Platelet-activating factor (PAF):

   a. Is an autacoid.
   b. Is an eicosanoid.
   c. Exerts its actions by stimulating G protein-linked cell surface receptors.
   d. Is a potent vasoconstrictor.
   e. Requires the presence of thromboxane$_2$ (TXA$_2$) to cause platelet aggregation.

4.36 An increase in the plasma concentration of the following generally leads to vasodilatation:

   a. Magnesium.
   b. Potassium.
   c. Acetate.
   d. Hydrogen ions.
   e. Endothelin.

4.37 The transmembranal transport of glucose can be effected by the following mechanisms:

   a. Simple diffusion.
   b. Facilitated diffusion.
   c. Primary active transport.
   d. Secondary active transport.
   e. Pinocytosis.

4.38 The following are pro-drugs:

   a. Enalapril.
   b. Diamorphine.
   c. Terbutaline.
   d. Valdecoxib.
   e. Oxazepam.

4.39 The following are physiological anticoagulants:

   a. Heparan.
   b. Nitric oxide.
   c. PGI$_2$.
   d. Plasmin.
   e. Thromboxane A$_2$.

4.40 Warfarin:

   a. Is a semi-synthetic anticoagulant.
   b. In its formulation for clinical use is a racemic mixture.
   c. Is only effective in vivo.
   d. In its action behaves as a competitive antagonist.
   e. Is metabolised mainly in the liver.

4.41 Insulin:

a. Is necessary for the entry of glucose into brain cells.
b. Activates the Na^+– K^+–ATPase pump.
c. Stimulates NO synthesis.
d. Increases renal sodium absorption.
e. Enhances glucagon secretion.

4.42 Non-depolarising neuromuscular blocking agents:

a. Are all quaternary ammonium compounds.
b. Are non-competitive blockers.
c. Need to bind to both α subunits of the receptor to produce their effects.
d. Possess some intrinsic agonist activity.
e. Can also act to block pre-synaptic acetylcholine receptors.

4.43 The following neuromuscular blocking agents are dependent, partly at least, on plasma esterases for their inactivation:

a. Atracurium.
b. Mivacurium.
c. Rocuronium.
d. Suxamethonium.
e. Vecuronium.

4.44 The following neuromuscular blocking agents on in vivo breakdown produce active metabolites:

a. Suxamethonium.
b. *Cis*-atracurium.
c. Mivacurium.
d. Pancuronium.
e. Rapacuronium.

4.45 Neostigmine:

a. Is a quaternary ammonium compound.
b. Owes its duration of action to its binding with the anionic site of acetylcholinesterase.
c. Inhibits plasma cholinesterase.
d. Can have a direct agonist action at nicotinic skeletal muscle junctions.
e. Can reverse the action of suxamethonium.

4.46 The following will enhance the accuracy and reliability of performance of a peripheral nerve stimulator:

a. Lower skin temperature of site of application of electrodes.
b. Placement of negative electrode close to nerve.
c. Increasing current strength to 100 mA.
d. Increasing pulse width to more than 1.0 ms.
e. Using a constant voltage rather than a constant current.

4.47 The following are reliable clinical indicators of recovery from neuromuscular blockade:

a. Ability to open eyes.
b. Sustained head lift for 5 seconds.
c. Sustained hand grip for 5 seconds.
d. Ability to phonate.
e. Ability to create an inspiratory pressure gradient of 40 cm H$_2$O.

4.48 The following statins (HMGCoA reductase inhibitors) are pro-drugs.

a. Atorvastatin.
b. Fluvastatin.
c. Lovastatin.
d. Pravastatin.
e. Simvastatin

4.49 In the case of glucocorticoids:

a. They are produced in the zona reticularis of the adrenal cortex.
b. They are stored for some time before release into the circulation.
c. They are highly bound to plasma proteins.
d. Their actions are mediated through cytoplasmic receptors.
e. They are inactivated in the liver.

4.50 Cimetidine:

a. Is a furan derivative.
b. Crosses the blood–brain barrier.
c. Can cause a bradycardia.
d. Inhibits alcohol dehydrogenase.
e. Has been known to cause impotence.

4.51 **The following are true with respect to the chemistry of induction anaesthetic agents:**

a. Thiopentone has a basic pyrimidine structure.
b. Methohexitone is a malonylurea derivative.
c. Propofol is a derivative of an aromatic alcohol.
d. Ketamine is a piperidine derivative.
e. Etomidate has the same basic structure as histamine.

4.52 **The hypnotic effect of thiopentone is owed to its:**

a. Basic barbiturate ring.
b. Sulphur substitution.
c. Side chain trunks.
d. Side chain radicals.
e. Marked alkalinity.

4.53 **Propofol:**

a. Is 3,6 di-isopropyl phenol.
b. Is light sensitive.
c. Is insoluble in water.
d. Is stable at room temperature.
e. Is compatible with 5% glucose solution.

4.54 **Etomidate:**

a. Is a benzyl-isoquinoline derivative.
b. Contains propylene glycol to render it water soluble.
c. Has been known to cause haemolysis.
d. May prolong the action of suxamethonium.
e. Is definitely contraindicated in patients with porphyria.

4.55 **Each of the following agents is presented for use as a mixture of two isomers, both of which have hypnotic properties:**

a. Thiopentone.
b. Methohexitone.
c. Propofol.
d. Ketamine.
e. Etomidate.

4.56 **Of the inhalational anaesthetic agents halothane, enflurane, isoflurane, sevoflurane and desflurane:**

a. Desflurane has the highest molecular weight.
b. Sevoflurane has the lowest biotransformation.
c. Halothane has the highest blood-gas partition coefficient.
d. Isoflurane has the lowest MAC.
e. Enflurane has the highest vapour pressure at room temperature.

4.57 Sevoflurane:

    a. Is a chiral agent.
    b. Has a blood-gas partition coefficient comparable with that of desflurane.
    c. Undergoes biotransformation to a lesser extent than isoflurane.
    d. Is not known to produce carbon monoxide with soda lime in low-flow systems.
    e. Is the only inhalational halogenated anaesthetic agent reputed to produce Compound A with soda lime.

4.58 Xenon:

    a. Is the only noble gas that is anaesthetic under normobaric conditions.
    b. Has a lower blood-gas partition coefficient than any currently used inhalational anaesthetic agent.
    c. Undergoes no known biotransformation.
    d. Is safe in the first trimester of pregnancy.
    e. Is best avoided in patients susceptible to malignant hyperpyrexia.

4.59 Oxygen:

    a. Is a polar molecule.
    b. Can be assayed by infra-red analysis.
    c. Is capable of two allotropic forms.
    d. In its gaseous state is repelled by regions of high magnetic flux.
    e. When oxygenating haemoglobin causes the displacement of water from the latter molecule.

4.60 The following gases are paramagnetic:

    a. Oxygen.
    b. Nitrogen dioxide.
    c. Nitric oxide.
    d. Nitrous oxide.
    e. Carbon dioxide.

4.61 The following may be found as additives in local anaesthetic preparations:

    a. Sodium metabisulphite.
    b. Thymol.
    c. Dextrose.
    d. Carbonate.
    e. *o*-toluidine.

4.62 The following statements are correct with respect to opioid analgesics:

a. Morphine is an endogenous opioid in the brain.
b. Remifentanil produces metabolites that are themselves analgesics.
c. Norpethidine has an analgesic action apart from its propensity to cause muscle rigidity.
d. Codeine has a better oral-parenteral potency ratio than morphine.
e. Naloxone is an antagonist at all opioid receptors.

4.63 Methadone:

a. Is a piperidine derivative.
b. Is structurally similar to propoxyphene.
c. Is primarily a μ agonist.
d. Owes its analgesic action essentially to its d-racemate.
e. Has a higher rate of renal excretion with an alkaline diuresis.

4.64 The respiratory depression of morphine:

a. Is due to direct depression of the respiratory centre in the medulla.
b. Is a $μ_1$ phenomenon.
c. Is mediated essentially by reduced responsiveness to CO_2.
d. Has a ceiling effect.
e. May be worsened by oxygen administration.

4.65 $GABA_B$ receptors are:

a. Present in high concentration in the dorsal horn cells of the spinal cord.
b. Present in pre-synaptic sites on peripheral autonomic terminals.
c. Essentially excitatory neuroreceptors.
d. Responsible for the actions of benzodiazepines.
e. The agonist site for baclofen.

4.66 Flumazenil:

a. Is structurally related to the benzodiazepines.
b. Is a competitive antagonist at benzodiazepine receptors.
c. Acts by altering the allosteric effects of benzodiazepines.
d. Antagonises the inverse agonist effects of benzodiazepines.
e. Is useful as an antagonist for single overdoses of tricyclic antidepressants.

4.67 Ingestion of aspirin can lead to the following acidoses:

   a. Of salicylic acid.
   b. Of lactic acid.
   c. Of acetoacetic acid.
   d. Of sulphuric acid.
   e. Of phosphoric acid.

4.68 Aspirin is contraindicated in:

   a. Pregnancy.
   b. Glucose-6-phosphate dehydrogenase deficiency.
   c. The asthmatic who is steroid dependent.
   d. Nasal polyps.
   e. Urticaria.

4.69 Preparations of gelatin colloid solutions for IV administration:

   a. Have a pH very near that of plasma.
   b. Have a higher water binding capacity than does albumin.
   c. Act as plasma substitutes by drawing water from the
      interstitial compartment to the intravascular compartment.
   d. Have no apparent effects on blood coagulation.
   e. Are eliminated essentially by metabolism.

Practice paper 4

4.70   The following are SI units:

a. Electron-volt (eV).
b. Torr.
c. Gray.
d. Gauss.
e. Cubic centimetre (cc).

4.71   The following have a direct linear relationship:

a. The partial pressure of a gas in a liquid and the number of moles of the gas dissolved in it.
b. The volume change of a fixed mass of gas and its celsius temperature, at a constant pressure.
c. The variation of saturated vapour pressure of an inhalational anaesthetic agent with temperature.
d. The variation of electrical conductance of a conductor with its kelvin temperature.
e. The viscosity of blood and its haematocrit.

4.72   The unit stated against each of the following physical phenomena is correct:

a. Strain: newtons per square metre.
b. Kinematic viscosity: pascal seconds.
c. Flow: litres.
d. Pulmonary elastance: centimetres of water per litre.
e. Current density (in relation to diathermy): amperes per square centimetre.

4.73   The following are graded according to French catheter gauge (FCG):

a. Epidural catheter.
b. Pulmonary artery flotation catheter.
c. Tracheal suction catheter.
d. Urinary catheter.
e. Quadruple central venous catheter.

4.74   The following devices measure temperature by measuring a dimensional change in matter:

a. Mercury clinical thermometer.
b. Alcohol thermometer.
c. Gas thermometer.
d. Bimetallic strip thermometer.
e. Bourdon gauge thermometer.

4.75 **The following when graphically represented take the form of a sine wave:**

    a. Variation with time of the mains AC voltage.
    b. Propagation of electromagnetic radiations.
    c. Energy discharge from a defibrillator.
    d. Current energy of a TOF stimulus from a PNS.
    e. Waves of a laser light beam.

4.76 **A high natural resonant frequency in an invasive arterial blood pressure monitoring system is achieved if:**

    a. A stiffer transducer diaphragm is used.
    b. A smaller volume dome is used.
    c. The system shows high compliance.
    d. The catheter length is increased.
    e. The indwelling cannula has a smaller cross-sectional area.

4.77 **According to international convention the shoulders of medical gas cylinders are coloured as follows:**

    a. Oxygen: alternating black and white.
    b. Helium 80% and oxygen 20%: brown.
    c. 5% CO_2 in oxygen: black and white.
    d. Nitrogen: black.
    e. Air: grey and black.

4.78 **The following cylinders, no matter their size, have a gas pressure of approximately 137 bar when full:**

    a. Oxygen.
    b. Nitrous oxide.
    c. Air.
    d. Helium–oxygen: 79%: 21%.
    e. Entonox.

4.79 **The Bodok seal on an anaesthetic machine can correctly be made of the following:**

    a. Wood.
    b. Fibre glass.
    c. Cork.
    d. Neoprene.
    e. Aluminium.

4.80 The 'machine pressure relief valve' on an anaesthetic machine:

a. Must necessarily be positioned downstream of the flowmeter unit.
b. Helps to eliminate the 'pumping effect' of a TEC vaporiser.
c. Is designed to open at a pressure of c. 400 cm water.
d. Need not be installed on a machine that operates solely off the piped gas supply.
e. Is there primarily to protect the patient from barotrauma.

4.81 The behaviour of a 'fixed performance' oxygen mask is in accordance with the following:

a. Bernoulli phenomenon.
b. Venturi effect.
c. Law of conservation of mechanical energy.
d. Hagen–Poiseuille law for gas flow.
e. Coanda effect.

4.82 The electric current in the following situations is of the order of milliamperes:

a. The 'can-let-go' current of electrocution.
b. The current that usually causes ventricular fibrillation.
c. The current conventionally used for transurethral resection of the prostate gland.
d. The current used to elicit TOF with a peripheral nerve stimulator.
e. The current used in conventional electroconvulsive therapy.

4.83 The following are higher in the newborn, compared with the young adult:

a. V_D/V_T ratio.
b. Alveolar ventilation per kilogram of body mass.
c. Blood volume per kilogram body mass.
d. The P_{50} haemoglobin.
e. Total body water as a percentage of body mass.

4.84 The following agents are known to accumulate in low-flow breathing attachments as a result of reaction between carbon dioxide and soda lime:

a. Methane.
b. Nitrogen peroxide.
c. Nitrogen.
d. Formic acid.
e. Water.

4.85 The 'pumping effect' of a plenum vaporiser is increased if the following are lower rather than higher:

a. Fresh gas flow rates.
b. Dial settings.
c. Level of liquid anaesthetic in the vaporiser chamber.
d. Respiratory rate.
e. Peak inspired pressures.

4.86 The following are recognised sources, phenomena or devices involved in the preparation of oxygen as a medical gas:

a. Joule–Kelvin effect.
b. Natural gas.
c. Adiabatic compression.
d. Brin process.
e. Zeolite.

4.87 The following breathing attachments are more 'efficient' than the co-axial Bain attachment for spontaneous ventilation:

a. Magill attachment.
b. Lack attachment.
c. Parallel Lack attachment.
d. Ayre's T-piece breathing attachment with Jackson Rees modification.
e. Waters' to-and-fro breathing attachment.

4.88 The following are 'rating' units, i.e. they indicate measurement of a quantity per unit time:

a. Watt.
b. Ampere.
c. Lumen.
d. Tesla.
e. Henry.

4.89 The following are correctly quantifiable in 'intensity' units, i.e. their activity is properly expressible in relation to unit surface area:

a. Pressure.
b. Surface tension.
c. Stress.
d. Illuminance.
e. Magnetic flux.

4.90 A newtonian fluid can be said to have the following properties:

a. A parabolic fluid flow profile.
b. A flow rate proportional to the square root of the pressure gradient.
c. A viscosity dependent on its flow rate.
d. A flow rate inversely proportional to the specific density of the fluid.
e. A flow rate proportional to the square of the cross-sectional area of the conduit.

4.1 Answers

a. **False** – beginning and end of the aortic arch.
b. **False** – the anterior end of the horizontal fissure of the right lung is at the 4th costochondral junction with the sternum. The Angle of Louis is at the junction of the anterior end of the 2nd rib with the sternum.
c. **True**.
d. **False** – the right recurrent laryngeal nerve hooks round the subclavian artery behind the right sternoclavicular joint.
e. **False** – the stellate ganglion lies in the interval between the transverse process of the 7th cervical vertebra and the neck of the 1st rib.

4.2 Answers

a. **False**.
b. **True**.
c. **False** – they are sparse.
d. **False** – they are absent, because they are responsible for active transport processes.
e. **False** – glial cells form a layer around the blood vessels of the brain but they do not form part of the blood–brain barrier itself.

4.3 Answers

a. **True**.
b. **True**.
c. **False** – they are all Type C.
d. **False** – dorsal column fibres cross in the brainstem.
e. **False** – pain, temperature and half of touch sensations travel in the anterolateral pathways, while pressure and the other half of touch sensations travel in the dorsal pathways.

4.4 Answers

a. **False** – remember the 'mantra': LR 6, SO 4, all the rest by 3': lateral rectus by the 6th (abducens), superior oblique by the 4th (trochlear), all the rest by the 3rd (oculomotor).
b. **True** – and runs in the 3rd cranial nerve.
c. **False** – in the 1st thoracic spinal segment.
d. **True** – it is partly sympathetic.
e. **True**.

4.5 Answers

a. **False** – it is the most posterior of all the openings and lies opposite the body of T12.
b. **True**.
c. **True** – because, of the aorta, oesophagus and the inferior vena cava, the latter is the most anterior of the three.
d. **True**.
e. **True**.

4.6 Answers

a. **False**.
b. **False** – it decreases with increasing distance from the heart. Note: the arterial pulse wave is taller and more peaked the further it is determined from the heart. Therefore the systolic pressure will be higher. However, because the diastolic pressure is lower and the duration of the pulse wave is shorter, the mean pressure is lower.
c. **False** – it is much higher because the aortic valve is closed and the pressure in the left ventricle has dropped.
d. **True** – because the mean pressure is determined by the area under the graph of a graphically displayed BP tracing.
e. **True** – the higher the heart rate, the shorter both systole and diastole, but diastole shortens disproportionately more. Therefore the systole–diastole ratio increases and other things being equal, the mean pressure must increase.

4.7 Answers

a. **True** – because the membrane of cells of the SA node is naturally leaky to sodium ions.
b. **True** – because of high permeability of its cell membranes as a result of the presence of gap junctions.
c. **True** – the phase of spontaneous repolarisation, plateau phase (phase 2).
d. **True** – neither has the ventricular musculature.
e. **False** – retrograde conduction is not normally possible in the AV node.

4.8 Answers

a. **False** – at 'postcapillary' venule.
b. **True** – of the blood volume of 5 L, c. 750–1000 ml is in the pulmonary circulation, c. 1500 ml is on the systemic arterial side, and the rest, c. 2500 ml, is in the veins.
c. **False** – the arterioles.
d. **False** – it depends also on the number of vessels in parallel.
e. **False** – they are wider at the venular end than at the arteriolar end.

4.9 Answers

a. **False** – they are about 7–8 μm thick.
b. **False** – the pulmonary capillaries contain only about 100 ml of blood at any time; the rest is divided about equally between the arteries and the veins.
c. **True**.
d. **False** – they inactivate noradrenaline (c. 30%), but not adrenaline.
e. **False** – they synthesise and release eicosanoids as required.

4.10 Answers

a. **True** – as well as Phase I biotransformation.
b. **False** – angiotensinogen, a plasma globulin made in the liver, is converted to angiotensin I in the plasma.
c. **True** – about 98% of 5-hydroxytryptamine is removed in a single pass through the pulmonary circulation, being taken up mainly by the capillary endothelium and then metabolised by mono-amine oxidase.
d. **True**.
e. **True**.

4.11 Answers

a. **False** – it is more abundant in infants and in fact is present in the fetus in the last trimester.
b. **True**.
c. **True** – β_1-adrenergic innervation. White fat has little direct sympathetic innervation, the principal innervation being to the blood vessels.
d. **True** – this must necessarily be so, as the mitochondria are the 'powerhouse' of the cells.
e. **True** – white fat mitochondria possess the usual inward proton conductance that generates ATP by oxidative phosphorylation. Brown fat has in addition a second proton conductance that does not generate ATP. This short circuit conductance is due to thermogenin, a polypeptide of MW 32 kD whose function is to cause an inward proton 'leak' that does not generate ATP. Consequently, metabolism of fat and generation of ATP are uncoupled, leading to energy release as heat.

4.12 Answers

a. **False** – it is a β_2-adrenergic effect.
b. **True**.
c. **False** – a decrease in insulin release.
d. **False** – it is an α_1 effect.
e. **False** – it is an α_1 effect.

4.13 Answers

a. **False** – situated just anterior to the coronary sinus ostium.
b. **False** – normally subject to vagal tone.
c. **False**.
d. **False** – it has a slower rate of spontaneous depolarisation than the SA node.
e. **True**.

4.14 Answers

a. **False** – its oxygen dissociation curve is a rectangular hyperbola.
b. **True** – because it is a single polypeptide chain attached to a single haem moiety. Compare haemoglobin, which has four haem moieties each attached to a globin chain and therefore binds four oxygen molecules per Hb molecule.
c. **True** – it is lower: c. 5 mmHg (0.67 kPa), compared with Hb, which is 27 mmHg (3.67 kPa).
d. **True**.
e. **True**.

4.15 Answers

a. **True** – c. 40 volumes per cent to oxygen's c. 20 volumes per cent.
b. **False**.
c. **False** – although the reaction can and does occur in the plasma it is a slow one. The several times (1000 ×) faster and more substantial reaction occurs in the red cells under the influence of carbonic anhydrase.
d. **True** – only about 0.0017 mol/L and accounts for less than 0.1% of the total CO_2 carriage.
e. **False** – 23% carbaminohaemoglobin: > 70% as bicarbonate; c. 7% as dissolved CO_2; and a very small percentage as carbonic acid (see **d**).

4.16 Answers

a. **False** – More than 60% of the albumin is in the interstitial space.
b. **True** – albumin MW 69,000. It is a single polypeptide chain of 585 amino acids folded into a series of α helices that form three structural domains and held together by 17 disulphide bonds.
c. **True**.
d. **True**.
e. **True**.

4.17 Answers

a. **True**.
b. **False** – also see answer to **e**.
c. **False** – angiotensin II is produced in the pulmonary circulation by conversion of angiotensin I by ACE.
d. **True**.
e. **True** – some 30% of noradrenaline is removed in a single first pass through the lungs. The difference in adrenaline and noradrenaline inactivation is not related to COMT or MAO levels but the result of selective uptake by the endothelium of noradrenaline.

4.18 Answers

a. **True**.
b. **True** – sodium is the predominant osmole of the plasma, and an increase in 1–2% of plasma osmolarity is sufficient to stimulate vasopressin release.
c. **True**.
d. **False** – alcohol inhibits vasopressin (ADH) release, one reason for an alcohol-induced diuresis.
e. **True**.

4.19 Answers

a. **True** – c. 2000 ml/minute per 100 g tissue.
b. **True** – Hering's nerve is the carotid body branch of the glossopharyngeal nerve.
c. **True** – but only at blood pressures below c. 80 mmHg.
d. **False** – the central chemoreceptors are about seven times more powerful.
e. **True** – about five times as much.

4.20 Answers

a. **True**.
b. **True** – lipases damage plasma membrane lipids, leading to release of arachidonic acid.
c. **True** – due to activation of NO synthase.
d. **True** – release of NO leads to production of peroxynitrite, which is a free radical that damages DNA.
e. **True** – the outcome of hypoxia.

4.21 Answers

a. **False**.
b. **True**.
c. **True**.
d. **False**.
e. **True**.

4.22 Answers

a. **True**.
b. **True**.
c. **False** – Zone 3 does.
d. **True**.
e. **False** – Zone 3 necrosis does.

4.23 Answers

a. **False** – Factor III is tissue thromboplastin.
b. **False** – Factor IV is calcium.
c. **False** – von Willebrand factor is synthesised in megakaryocytes and the vascular endothelium.
d. **True**.
e. **True**.

4.24 Answers

a. **False**.
b. **True**.
c. **False**.
d. **True** – it is a secondary active process dependent on sodium absorption down its concentration gradient. However, the converse is not true. Glucose absorption is only one process that determines Na^+ absorption and only prevails during the postprandial phase. During the interdigestive period other mechanisms are the primary determinants of Na^+ absorption.
e. **True**.

4.25 Answers

a. **True** – due to: (i) an increase in lactic acid production; and (ii) accumulation of fatty acids and ketone bodies.
b. **False** – it is inhibited, leading to hypoglycaemia.
c. **True**.
d. **False** – fatty acids cannot be oxidised; they are merely converted into ketone bodies.
e. **False** – it is reduced because the overproduction of lactic acid blocks renal excretion of uric acid.

4.26 Answers

a. **True** – the brain is normally dependent on glucose for > 90% of its metabolic substrate (c. 75 mg per minute) and on a small amount of glutamate (c. 5.6 mg per minute). But in conditions of severe starvation it can use ketones for up to 50% of its metabolic needs, the rest being met by glucose.

b. **True** – in fact under normal conditions the heart muscle cells utilise fats and ketones as part of their energy substrate.

c. **False** – the liver is the only organ that produces ketone bodies for metabolism by brain, heart, kidney and muscle, but it does not use this substrate for its own energy requirements.

d. **True**.

e. **False** – red cells are solely dependent on glucose as their sole metabolic substrate.

4.27 Answers

a. **True** – the Na^+–K^+–ATPase pump, by keeping sodium out of the cell, helps keep water out of the ICF and thus maintains its integrity.

b. **True** – by pumping out sodium at the basolateral border of the gut cell wall, the Na^+–K^+–ATPase pump maintains a sodium gradient from the intestinal lumen to the cell interior, thus enabling the absorption of sodium from the gut lumen. This gradient then acts as a co-transport mechanism for glucose absorption.

c. **True** – the mechanism is the same as for sodium–gluocse co-transport in the gut.

d. **True** – Digoxin inhibits the Na^+–K^+–ATPase pump. This leads to a higher level of Na^+ inside the cell, and then a diminished extracellular/intracellular Na^+ gradient results in slower extrusion of Ca^{2+} by the Na^+/Ca^{2+} exchanger. The consequent increase in intracellular Ca^{2+} enhances contractility of the cardiac muscle.

e. **False** – gastric acid secretion is effected by the H^+–K^+–ATPase pump, which is similar to the Na^+–K^+–ATPase pump (they are both members of the gene family of P-type ATPases), but the activity of the latter is not essential for the proper functioning of the former.

4.28 Answers

a. **False** – the intercostals too play a part, albeit a minor one.

b. **True** – the intrapleural pressure is always subatmospheric during quiet spontaneous ventilation.

c. **True**.

d. **False** – heat energy is lost in about equal amounts in the two phases of ventilation.

e. **True** – it is dependent on the elastic recoil of the lungs as a result of the potential energy stored in the chest wall and lungs during inspiration.

4.29 Answers

a. **False** – it is the other way round.
b. **True**.
c. **False** – Type II cells produce surfactant.
d. **False** – heparin is produced by the mast cells on the outside layer of the capillary endothelium.
e. **False** – ACE is produced by capillary endothelial cells.

4.30 Answers

a. **False** – the reciprocal of compliance is elastance. Resistance is the reciprocal of conductance.
b. **False** – it is the change in lung volume by the change in pressure at the end of inspiration, i.e. when ventilation has ceased, hence the term 'static'.
c. **True** – the lung volume change is very easily measured. The pressure change can be determined by oesophageal pressure measurement.
d. **False** – $1/C_{Total} = 1/C_{Lung} + 1/C_{Chest\ wall}$.
e. **False** – prolonged breathing of high O_2 concentrations will lead to alveolar collapse, which in turn will lead to a higher intra-alveolar pressure per unit increase in lung volume. Therefore compliance will be reduced.

4.31 Answers

a. **False** – angiotensin I is the decapeptide, which on being cleaved of two amino acids, histidine and leucine, becomes angiotensin II, an octapeptide.
b. **False** – the half-life is c.1–2 minutes.
c. **True** – c. 4–8 times as potent.
d. **False**.
e. **True** – by a direct action on the nerve endings.

4.32 Answers

a. **False** – it is a glycoprotein, consisting of 165 amino acids and four oligosaccharides.
b. **False** – 85% is produced in kidneys and c. 15% in liver.
c. **False** – the circulation $t_{1/2}$ is about 5 hours.
d. **True**.
e. **True**.

4.33 Answers

a. **True** – an amphiphilic substance is the same as an 'amphipathic' substance – it is both lipophilic and hydrophilic.
b. **True**.
c. **True**.
d. **True**.
e. **True**.

4.34 Answers

a. **True** – hence the term 'eicosanoids' because *eikosi* in Greek means 'twenty'.
b. **False** – they are usually unsaturated fatty acids with 3, 4 or 5 double bonds.
c. **False** – normally in *cis* form.
d. **True**.
e. **False** – SRS-A is in fact a mixture of LTC_4 and LTD_4 (leukotriene C_4 and leukotriene D_4), which are both eicosanoids.

4.35 Answers

a. **True** – 'autacoid' literally means 'self-remedy: *autos* ('self') *acos* ('remedy') and refer to agents that act at sites closeted from the general circulation, i.e. locally, as opposed to true hormones, which reach their sites of action via the bloodstream.
b. **False** – PAF is a modified phospholipid, not a 20-carbon fatty acid.
c. **True**.
d. **False** – PAF is a potent vasodilator.
e. **False** – PAF does not require TXA_2 to cause platelet aggregation, but is accompanied by the release of TXA_2 and granular contents from platelets.

4.36 Answers

a. **True**.
b. **True**.
c. **True** – one reason for the vasodilatation following alcohol consumption.
d. **True** – an acidosis causes vasodilatation.
e. **False** – endothelin released from damaged capillary endothelium causes vasoconstriction in an attempt to minimise bleeding.

4.37 Answers

a. **True** – a rare method, present at the basement membrane border of intestinal epithelium, which allows glucose to enter the capillaries.

b. **True** – by means of GLUT 1–5 (glucose transporter). They have slightly different amino acid compositions and their affinity for glucose varies. Their activity is enhanced by insulin. GLUT 4 is the one in muscle and adipose tissue, and is especially sensitive to insulin.

c. **False**.

d. **True** – by sodium-dependent glucose transporter (SGLT 1) – a co-transporter whose primary function is to transport Na^+ down its concentration gradient from the lumen into the cell in the intestine and the renal tubule. The energy gradient created by the sodium *secondarily* transports the glucose.

e. **False**.

4.38 Answers

a. **True** – it is hydrolysed to its dicarboxylic acid form, enalaprilat, which is the pharmacologically active agent.

b. **True** – it needs to be converted to morphine via 6-monoacetylmorphine to exert its effect as an opioid analgesic.

c. **False** – the pro-drug is bambuterol, which is converted to the active agent the β_2 agonist terbutaline.

d. **False** – the pro-drug is parecoxib, which is converted to its active moiety valdecoxib.

e. **False** – oxazepam is active in its own right and indeed is a metabolite of diazepam.

4.39 Answers

a. **True**. (Note: the allusion is to 'heparan', not 'heparin').

b. **True**.

c. **True**.

d. **True**.

e. **False**.

4.40 Answers

a. **True** – it is a modified coumarin derivative.

b. **True**.

c. **True** – because its activity is 'biological' and not merely 'chemical'.

d. **True** – it competes with vitamin K for the carboxyglutamate radicals of the coagulation factors.

e. **True**.

4.41 Answers

a. **False** – glucose enters brain cells via a glucose transporter found in high concentration in brain capillaries, which appears to be identical to the type I glucose transporter GLUT I found in erythrocytes.

Insulin is not a necessary agent, otherwise diabetics would suffer brain damage from hypoglycaemia early in their disease history. On the other hand, insulin hypoglycaemia can cause brain damage because insulin causes glucose to be removed rapidly from the ECF into general cells of the body. This is a more avid process compared with the brain's glucose transporter mechanism. This leads to the brain being severely starved of glucose.

b. **True** – this normally occurs in liver and muscle.
c. **True**.
d. **True** – partly by increasing the activity of the Na^+–K^+–ATPase pump at the basolateral membrane.
e. **False** – counteracts glucagon secretion.

4.42 Answers

a. **True** – so are depolarising blockers.
b. **False** – they are competitive blockers. Depolarising blockers are non-competitive blockers.
c. **False** – binding with one α subunit will suffice to bring about NM blockade.
d. **False**.
e. **True**.

4.43 Answers

a. **True** – atracurium is broken down: (i) by Hoffmann degradation: spontaneous non-enzymatic breakdown at physiological temperatures and pH; and (ii) by plasma esterases.
b. **True** – mivacurium is enzymatically degraded by butyryl cholinesterase.
c. **False** – rocuronium is eliminated primarily by the liver.
d. **True** – suxamethonium is hydrolysed by butyryl cholinesterase.
e. **False** – vecuronium is eliminated mainly by hepatic breakdown.

4.44 Answers

a. True – suxamethonium on hydrolysis is first broken down to succinyl monocholine, which has a weak neuromuscular blocking action.

b. False – although *cis*-atracurium produces laudanosine and acrylates, like atracurium does, none of the products possesses neuromuscular blocking activity.

c. False – mivacurium is hydrolysed by plasma pseudocholinesterase to inactive metabolites.

d. True – the 3-OH metabolite of pancuronium has approximately half the potency of the parent compound.

e. True – rapacuronium is broken down to its 3-desacetyl derivative, which too has neuromuscular blocking properties.

4.45 Answers

a. True – it owes its action to this attribute.

b. True – edrophonium owes its short-lasting effect to binding with the anionic site of the enzyme only. Neostigmine binds with both the anionic site and the esteratic site of the enzyme. The latter combination gives neostigmine a longer duration of action.

c. True.

d. True.

e. True – can effect partial reversal when there is Phase II block after prolonged suxamethonium administration.

4.46 Answers

a. False – the lower the skin temperature the greater the skin impedance and therefore a lower current in accordance with Ohm's law.

b. True.

c. False – use of a higher current may lead to direct stimulation of the muscle.

d. False.

e. False – it is current and not voltage that is the determinant of stimulation. A change in skin impedance with a constant voltage will change the current (according to Ohm's law) and thus the current energy required for the stimulus.

4.47 Answers

a. False.

b. True.

c. True.

d. False.

e. True.

4.48 Answers

a. **False**.
b. **False**.
c. **True** – it possesses a lactone ring that requires metabolism to β-hydroxyacid (open) form to be active.
d. **False**.
e. **True** – same as **c**.

4.49 Answers

a. **False** – the zona fasciculata of the adrenal cortex.
b. **False** – glucocorticoids are synthesised and released as required under the influence of ACTH.
c. **True** – c. 95% are bound to corticosteroid-binding globulin (CBG) and to albumin.
d. **True** – intracellular receptors belonging to the super family of receptors that control gene transcription.
e. **True**.

4.50 Answers

a. **False** – cimetidine is an imidazole derivative with a bulky side chain. Note: the imidazole ring is the main part of histamine. The furan ring is part of the structure of ranitidine.
b. **True**.
c. **True** – due to interaction with cardiac H_2 receptors.
d. **True** – therefore it enhances the action of alcohol.
e. **True**.

4.51 Answers

a. **True**.
b. **True** – this is the same as the pyrimidine nucleus (see **a**.)
c. **True** – it is a phenol substitute.
d. **False** – it is a phencyclidine derivative.
e. **True** – structurally they are both imidazoles.

4.52 Answers

a. **False**.
b. **False** – the sulphur atom confers rapidity of action and recovery.
c. **True**.
d. **True**.
e. **False**.

4.53 Answers

a. **False** – it is 2,6 di-isopropyl phenol.
b. **False**.
c. **True**.
d. **True**.
e. **True**.

4.54 Answers

a. **False** – it is an imidazole derivative.
b. **False** – etomidate is soluble in water. The propylene glycol improves stability and reduces local irritant effects.
c. **True** – due to the propylene glycol.
d. **True** – because of a slight depressant effect on pseudocholinesterase.
e. **False** – etomidate inhibits d-aminolaevulinic acid synthetase in vitro, but it has not been known to provoke an attack of porphyria in susceptible persons.

4.55 Answers

a. **True** – the S (*l*) isomer is roughly twice as potent as the R (*d*) isomer.
b. **True** – same as **a**.
c. **False** – propofol is an achiral compound.
d. **True** – but the S (+) isomer is more potent (and has fewer side effects).
e. **False** – etomidate exists as two isomers but only the (+) isomer is active as a hypnotic.

4.56 Answers

a. **False** – sevoflurane: 200; desflurane: 168; halothane: 197; enflurane: 184.5; isoflurane: 184.5.
b. **False** – desflurane: 0.02%; halothane: 20–25%; enflurane: 2–2.5%; isoflurane: 0.2–0.25%; sevoflurane c. 3–3.5%.
c. **True** – halothane: 2.3; enflurane: 1.8; isoflurane: 1.4; sevoflurane: 0.65; desflurane: 0.45.
d. **False** – isoflurane: 1.2; halothane: 0.75; enflurane: 1.6; sevoflurane: 2.0; desflurane: 6.0.
e. **False** – desflurane: 669 mmHg; halothane: 243; enflurane: 175; isoflurane: 250; sevoflurane: 160.

4.57 **Answers**

a. **False** – the only achiral inhalational halogenated anaesthetic agent.
b. **True** – desflurane: c. 0.47; sevoflurane: 0.6.
c. **False** – isoflurane: c. 0.2–0.25; sevoflurane: c. 3–3.5.
d. **True** – because it does not possess a $-CHF_2$ moiety. It has a $-CH_2F$ moiety.
e. **True**.

4.58 **Answers**

a. **True**.
b. **True** – 0.115.
c. **True**.
d. **True** – it is non-teratogenic.
e. **False** – is not reputed to cause malignant hyperpyrexia.

4.59 **Answers**

a. **False** – the molecule of oxygen, having as it does just two identical oxygen atoms, cannot exhibit polarity as between the two atoms. Therefore it is non-polar.
b. **False** – for an agent to be capable of assay by infra-red analysis it must have at least two dissimilar atoms in its molecule.
c. **True** – oxygen and ozone. Allotopic forms of an element exist in the same state (gaseous in the case of oxygen and ozone) but in more than one structural form. They have the same or similar chemical properties but their physical properties are different because each allotrope has its own crystal structure. Other allotropes include carbon, sulphur, phosphorus, tin and lead.
d. **False** – it is attracted towards regions of high magnetic flux, i.e. it is paramagnetic, a property it owes to the presence of an unpaired electron.
e. **True** – when oxygen combines with haemoglobin it displaces a molecule of water from the Fe^{2+} of haem iron.

4.60 Answers

a. **True**.
b. **True**.
c. **True**.
d. **False**.
e. **False**.

The property of paramagnetism is dependent on the presence of 'unpaired electrons' in the outer shell of the atom of the gas. According to Pauli's Exclusion Principle, paired electrons in the same orbit must possess oppositely directed electrons and hence their magnetic moments cancel out each other. The presence of unpaired electrons means there is a magnetic moment and thus paramagnetism. Oxygen has two unpaired electrons in its outer shell.

Wolfgang Ernst Pauli (1900–1958) won the Nobel prize for physics in 1945.

4.61 Answers

a. **True** – as a reducing agent so as to prevent oxidation of the agent.
b. **True** – it acts as a fungicide.
c. **True** – to render bupivacaine hyperbaric ('heavy' bupivacaine) for use as spinals.
d. **True** – to render the agent alkaline and thus hasten absorption and onset of action.
e. **False** – o-toluidine is a metabolite of prilocaine that is responsible for methaemoglobinaemia with that agent.

4.62 Answers

a. **True**.
b. **False** – its metabolites are, to all practical purposes, inactive.
c. **True**.
d. **True** – 60%, compared with 25% for morphine.
e. **True**.

4.63 Answers

a. **False**.
b. **True**.
c. **True**.
d. **False** – to its l- racemate.
e. **False** – with an acid diuresis.

4.64 Answers

a. **True**.
b. **False** – it is a μ_2 phenomenon. μ_1 receptors are responsible for supraspinal analgesia.
c. **True**.
d. **False** – it is dose related.
e. **True**.

4.65 Answers

a. **True**.
b. **True**.
c. **False** – their activity diminishes the release of neurotransmitters.
d. **False** – benzodiazepines act via $GABA_A$ receptors.
e. **True**.

4.66 Answers

a. **True** – it is an imidazobenzodiazepine.
b. **True**.
c. **True** – does so in addition to altering the primary effect of benzodiazepines.
d. **True**.
e. **False**.

4.67 Answers

a. **True** – because aspirin on hepatic first-pass metabolism is broken down into salicylic acid.
b. **True** – because in overdosage it can lead to anaerobic metabolism and a buildup of lactic acid (and pyruvic acid).
c. **True** – because it can cause derangement of carbohydrate metabolism, which leads to formation of ketone bodies, of which acetoacetic acid is one (the other two are acetone and β-hydroxy butyric acid).
d. **True** – renal failure from aspirin overdosage can lead to the accumulation of sulphuric acid.
e. **True** – for the same reasons as in **d**.

4.68 Answers

a. **False**.
b. **True** – because of its tendency to cause haemolysis.
c. **True**.
d. **True**.
e. **True**.

4.69 Answers

a. **True**.
b. **False** – water binding capacity: gelatins: 15 ml/g; albumin: 18 ml/g; HESs: 20–30 ml/g.
c. **False** – act as plasma substitutes by being retained in the plasma compartment, thereby maintaining the intravascular fluid volume.
d. **True**.
e. **False** – only c. 1–3% is metabolised.

4.70 Answers

a. **False** – an electron-volt is the energy equal to the work done on an electron in moving it through a potential difference of 1 V. The corresponding SI unit is the joule. One eV = 1.602×10^{-19} J.
b. **False** – 1 Torr is almost equal to 1 mmHg pressure.
c. **True** – a derived SI unit, the gray is the unit of absorbed dose of ionising radiation, i.e. the absorbed dose when the energy per unit mass imparted to matter by ionising radiation is 1 J/kg.
d. **False** – the gauss is the CGS unit of magnetic flux density and has been replaced by the tesla, which is equal to 10,000 gauss.
e. **False** – the equivalent SI unit is 10^{-6} of a cubic metre, commonly called a 'millilitre'.

4.71 Answers

a. **True** – this is in effect Henry's law.
b. **True** – this is in effect Charles' law and the change is the same, be it the kelvin scale or the celsius scale.
c. **False** – the change is an 'accelerating growth exponential' curve.
d. **False** – the change is one of inverse relationship.
e. **False** – the change is an 'accelerating growth exponential' curve.

4.72 Answers

a. **False** – strain is a dimensionless entity; it has no units, as it indicates a ratio:change of length (for instance) per unit original length.
b. **False** – kinematic viscosity is dynamic viscosity divided by density (of the fluid concerned): η/ρ ; the dimensional formula for kinematic viscosity is $[L]^2 [T]^{-1}$, i.e. metres squared per second. The CGS unit of kinematic viscosity is the stokes (St).
c. **False** – 'flow' in the context of fluids is a rating and therefore the units are 'litres per unit time' (second/minute).
d. **True** – it is the reciprocal of compliance, the units of which are litres per cm water.
e. **False** – it is watts per square centimetre.

4.73 Answers

a. **False** – according to steel wire gauge (SWG).
b. **True** – integrates 4 lumens into a 7 F catheter.
c. **True**.
d. **True**.
e. **False** – according to SWG.

Note: FCG is a unit with dimensions. It is the external circumference of the device in millimetres. SWG has no dimensions. It refers to the number of the particular device that can be accommodated in a standard measuring device. For this reason the higher the SWG number the smaller the bore of the device. Example: cannulae.

4.74 Answers

a. **True** – by measuring the increase in volume (dimensional change) of the mercury as a result of expansion.
b. **True** – same as **a**.
c. **True** – same as **a** and **b**.
d. **True** – expansion of the metal strip (dimensional change) leads to deflection of the pointer on the scale.
e. **False** – expansion of the gas puts tension on the hollow tube, causing it to 'unfurl' and thereby move a pointer on a scale, just as in the Bourdon pressure gauge of a gas cylinder.

4.75 Answers

a. **True**.
b. **True**.
c. **False** – the traditional discharge was a decelerating exponential decay. Later it had a 'damped sine wave' configuration. Modern defibrillators can now discharge the current energy as monophasic or biphasic and also in a 'saw tooth', 'rectilinear' and 'truncated' manner.
d. **False** – it is a square wave.
e. **True** – laser light, like ordinary light, is propagated as a sine wave.

4.76 Answers

a. **True**.
b. **True**.
c. **False** – the system will resonate better with low compliance.
d. **False**.
e. **False**.

4.77 Answers

a. **False** – white, with a black body.
b. **False** – the body is black, the shoulder is brown and white.
c. **False** – white and grey, with a black body.
d. **False** – the body is black, the shoulder is grey.
e. **False** – the body is grey, the shoulder is black and white.

4.78 Answers

a. **True**.
b. **False** – a 'full' nitrous oxide cylinder has a pressure of about 45 bar.
c. **True**.
d. **True**.
e. **True**.

4.79 Answers

a. **False**.
b. **False**.
c. **False**.
d. **True**.
e. **True**.

Note: the Bodok seal must be capable of withstanding high pressures and therefore adiabatic compression, which when it occurs causes a rise in temperature from heat production. Therefore any material in the vicinity must be non-flammable.

4.80 Answers

a. **True**.
b. **False** – the pumping effect will be seen at a lower pressure than that which opens the relief valve.
c. **True**.
d. **False**.
e. **False** – it is there primarily to protect the machine. A pressure of 400 cm water is far too high a pressure for the lungs to withstand.

4.81 Answers

a. **True**.
b. **True**.
c. **True**.
d. **False**.
e. **False**.

4.82 Answers

a. **True** – it is about 10–15 mA.
b. **True** – about 80–100 mA.
c. **False** – of the order of about 1.5–2 A.
d. **True** – about 60 mA.
e. **True** – 100 to c. 900 mA.

4.83 Answers

a. **False** – the ratio is about the same: 0.3. V_D; c. 5 ml V_T; c. 16 ml.
b. **True** – adult: c. 60 ml/kg; newborn: c. 100–150 ml/kg.
c. **True** – newborn: c. 80–85 ml/kg; adult: c. 70–75 ml/kg.
d. **False** – newborn: 20 mmHg, 2.6 kPa; adult: 27 mmHg, 3.8 kPa.
e. **True** – newborn: c. 70%; adult: c. 60%.

4.84 Answers

a. **False** – methane accumulates but because it is exhaled by the patient.
b. **False**: minute amounts of nitrogen peroxide accumulate because it is a 'contaminant' present in nitrous oxide, but it is not as a result of reaction of CO_2 with soda lime.
c. **False** – nitrogen is present because it is exhaled by the patient.
d. **True** – as a by-product in the formation of CO by sevoflurane by the 'cannizzaro disproportionation reaction'.
e. **True** – water is a by-product of the reaction between CO_2 and soda lime.

4.85 Answers

a. **True**.
b. **True**.
c. **True** – because there is more space above the liquid surface for the carrier gases.
d. **False** – it is increased if the respiratory rate is higher.
e. **False**.

4.86 Answers

a. **True** – also known as the Joule–Thomson effect (because Sir William Thomson was later Lord Kelvin), it is the cooling effect following adiabatic expansion of a gas, a method employed in the production of oxygen by the process of fractional distillation of air.

b. **False** – natural gas is the main source of helium. Oxygen is not obtained from natural gas.

c. **False** – it is adiabatic expansion (see **a** above).

d. **True** – now obsolete, the Brin process involved exposing barium oxide to air at a temperature of 700°C and 2 atmospheres pressure, which converted the BaO_2 to barium peroxide and then reducing the pressure to 0.05 bar, when the peroxide reverted to BaO_2, releasing the oxygen.

e. **True** – 'zeolite' literally means *boiling stone* (Greek: zeein: boil; lithos: stone), a term coined in 1756 by the Swedish scientist Baron Cronstedt, who discovered a mineral which appeared to boil and release steam when heated. Zeolites are a family of aluminium silicates that contain a network of channels, rather like those in a sponge. These channels, depending on their size, will permit smaller molecules to go through but trap larger molecules. This is the 'molecular sieve' basis of separating oxygen from the rest of the ingredients of air.

4.87 Answers

a. **True**.
b. **True**.
c. **True**.
d. **False**.
e. **True**.

Note: the 'efficiency' of an anaesthetic breathing attachment is gauged by the ratio of the fresh gas flow rate to the minute volume, which will maintain normocapnia. In this respect the order, starting with the most efficient is: parallel Lack, Magill, Waters', co-axial Bain and Ayre's T-piece.

4.88 Answers

a. **True** – watts = joules per second.

b. **True** – amperes = coulombs per second.

c. **True** – lumens = candela per second per steradian.

d. **False** – tesla = webers per square metre.

e. **True** – henry: the unit of inductance. It is that inductance (as a back EMF of 1 V) that results in a coil when the current in it changes at a rate of 1 A/second.

4.89 Answers

a. **True** – pressure is force per unit area.

b. **True** – surface tension is force per unit length (i.e. newtons per metre), which is the same as 'energy per unit area (joules per square metre).

c. **True** – the units of stress are the same as those of pressure: newtons per square metre.

d. **True** – illuminance is the amount of light actually shining on a surface and is expressed in lumens per square metre.

e. **False** – magnetic flux is expressed in webers. Magnetic flux density is the 'intensity' unit and is expressed in tesla, i.e. webers per square metre.

4.90 Answers

a. **True**.

b. **False** – the flow rate is proportional to the pressure gradient, because if the fluid is newtonian its flow is laminar and it obeys the Hagen–Poiseuille equation. It is when flow is turbulent that the flow rate is proportional to the square root of the pressure gradient.

c. **False** – in laminar flow (see **b** above) viscosity is constant.

d. **False** – density plays no part in laminar flow.

e. **True** – cross-sectional area^2 = radius^4. Note: this is only a mathematical notion and is not possible in reality.

Practice paper 5

Anatomy

5.1 **In the case of the brachial plexus:**

a. It is formed solely from the ventral rami of spinal nerves.
b. It is solely responsible for the cutaneous nerve supply of the upper limb.
c. It provides the sole motor supply to all the muscles acting on the upper limb.
d. None of its cords receives contributions from all five ventral rami.
e. None of its motor nerve supply to muscles originates 'upstream' of its divisions.

5.2 **The oculomotor nerve:**

a. Is the only one of the first six cranial nerves to carry parasympathetic fibres.
b. Enters the orbit as a single nerve.
c. Supplies all the intrinsic muscles of the eye except the lateral rectus muscle.
d. Conveys fibres from the Edinger–Westphal nucleus.
e. Conveys fibres to the sphincter pupillae muscle.

5.3 **Capillary endothelial 'tight junctions' are a distinctive feature of the following:**

a. Blood–brain barrier.
b. Feto-maternal vascular interface.
c. Pulmonary alveolar capillary endothelium.
d. Luminal surface of the small intestinal epithelium.
e. Cellular lining of the renal tubule.

5.4 **The inguinal region receives its cutaneous sensory supply from the following spinal nerves:**

a. T10.
b. T11.
c. T12.
d. L1.
e. L2.

5.5 The following are anatomical differences between the thoracic and lumbar vertebrae:

a. The thoracic column is concave forwards, while the lumbar column is concave backwards.
b. The thoracic intervertebral foramina are circular while the lumbar intervertebral foramina are triangular.
c. Each thoracic vertebral body is roughly cylindrical, while each lumbar vertebral body is wider in the coronal plane compared with the sagittal plane.
d. The thoracic vertebrae increase in size progressively from top downwards, while the lumbar are approximately all the same.
e. The thoracic spines incline downwards and backwards, while the lumbar spines project horizontally backwards.

Physiology

5.6　In the case of the arterial wave produced by the ejection of the left ventricular stroke volume:

a. The amplitude of its pressure pulse wave decreases as it travels away from the heart.
b. Its wavefront becomes steeper.
c. Its dicrotic notch is accentuated.
d. Its two components, pressure pulse wave and blood flow, travel down the arterial tree at the same velocity.
e. Its waveform can be augmented by wave reflections.

5.7　During normal cardiac activity:

a. The ejection fraction at rest is about 60–70%.
b. The energy substrate for muscle contraction is almost entirely glucose.
c. The maximum efficiency of the normal heart is of the order of 70–75%.
d. Atrial contraction only accounts for about 25% of ventricular filling.
e. The higher the heart rate the lower the ratio of duration of systole to duration of diastole.

5.8　The right atrium:

a. Normally contracts slightly earlier than the left.
b. Normally is at a pressure of slightly above 0 mmHg.
c. Can have a 'negative' pressure inside it if the heart were to pump very forcefully.
d. Plays a role in the activity of the Bainbridge reflex.
e. Is the sole cardiac chamber for producing atrial natriuretic peptide.

5.9　The following are phenomena associated with cardiac ventricular activity:

a. Bezold–Jarisch reflex.
b. Starling phenomenon.
c. Stress–relaxation.
d. Latch bridge mechanism.
e. Paul Bert effect.

5.10 Concerning the generation sites of the cardiac action potential:

a. Impulse conduction is slowest in the Bundle of His.
b. The AV bundle is the only part where retrograde conduction is normally not possible.
c. The sodium current (I_{Na}) is not present in the sinoatrial and atrioventricular nodes.
d. The Purkinje fibres have the lowest intrinsic pacemaker rate.
e. The ventricular musculature has no time-dependent currents during phase 4.

5.11 In the systemic circulation:

a. More than 50% of the vascular resistance lies in the arterioles.
b. Approximately 50% of the blood volume is normally located in the arterial tree.
c. Velocity of pressure pulse transmission is directly related to vessel wall compliance.
d. Mean arterial pressure at all ages is nearer the diastolic than the systolic pressure.
e. Colloid osmotic pressure is a direct linear function of the plasma protein concentration.

5.12 When measuring blood pressure using a mercury sphygmomanometer and the auscultation method:

a. The zero reference point of the mercury scale ought to be at the level of the arm cuff.
b. A faster rate of cuff deflation gives a falsely higher systolic pressure reading.
c. The slower the heart rate the less the error in the reading.
d. More correct values are obtained if a cuff with a single connecting tube is used.
e. It suffices to have a cuff with a width just equal to the diameter of the arm it is applied to.

5.13 Haem is an integral moiety of the following:

a. Myoglobin.
b. Cytochrome oxidase.
c. Bilirubin.
d. Protoporphyrin.
e. Guanylyl cyclase.

5.14 **Myoglobin:**

   a. Is a tetramer.
   b. Acts as an oxygen transporter.
   c. Has a higher P_{50} than fetal haemoglobin.
   d. Has an oxygen dissociation curve that is a rectangular hyperbola.
   e. Is poisoned by carbon monoxide.

5.15 **When oxygen combines with haemoglobin:**

   a. The combination is enzyme dependent.
   b. The oxygen combines with the Fe^{2+} of the haem moiety by covalent linkage.
   c. The combination can correctly be called an allosteric reaction.
   d. One molecule of oxygen combines with one molecule of haemoglobin.
   e. The globin chains move closer to each other in the process.

5.16 **The combination of CO_2 with haemoglobin to form carbaminohaemoglobin:**

   a. Is an enzyme-dependent process.
   b. Is a faster reaction than that between CO_2 and water inside red cells to form H_2CO_3.
   c. Occurs with the Fe^{2+} ions of the haem moiety.
   d. Results in the globin chains of haemoglobin moving nearer each other.
   e. Leads to the Haldane effect.

5.17 **An increase in concentration of red cell 2,3 DPG (diphosphoglycerate) is associated with:**

   a. A rise in cell pH.
   b. A fall in P_{50}.
   c. A rise in blood thyroxine levels.
   d. A fall in body temperature.
   e. A rise in carbaminohaemoglobin.

5.18 **Prostaglandins have the following functions:**

   a. Stimulation of inflammation.
   b. Regulation of blood flow to particular organs.
   c. Control of ion transport across membranes.
   d. Modulation of synaptic transmission.
   e. Induction of sleep.

5.19 The breakdown of the following is catalysed by MAO (monoamine oxidase):

a. Adrenaline.
b. Ephedrine.
c. Acetylcholine.
d. Serotonin (5-hydroxytryptamine).
e. Histamine.

5.20 Vasopressin (ADH):

a. Is an octapeptide.
b. Is structurally very similar to oxytocin.
c. Causes hepatic glycogenolysis.
d. Stimulates ACTH secretion by the anterior pituitary.
e. Owes its antidiuretic action to its mediation at V_{1A} receptors.

5.21 Brown adipose tissue ('brown fat'):

a. Is more likely to be present in obese persons.
b. Contains thermogenin.
c. Produces more ATP than other tissues.
d. Shows less coupling of oxidation and phosphorylation than 'white' fat.
e. Shows a marked proton gradient across the inner membrane of its mitochondria.

5.22 Consumption of alcohol leads to an increase in urine production by the following mechanisms:

a. An increase in fluid load.
b. An osmotic diuretic effect of alcohol.
c. Inhibition of ADH secretion.
d. Decrease in aldosterone production.
e. Direct suppression of ANP.

5.23 Endothelin 1:

a. Is a nonapeptide.
b. Is a vasodilator.
c. Has a half-life of 1–2 minutes.
d. Is inactivated during its passage through the pulmonary circulation.
e. Is offset by NO with respect to its effect on blood vessels.

5.24 Compared with arterial blood, mixed venous blood has:

    a. A higher haematocrit.
    b. A lower pH.
    c. Slightly larger red cells.
    d. A lower plasma chloride concentration.
    e. A higher total gas pressure.

5.25 During normal quiet spontaneous ventilation:

    a. The diaphragm is the sole muscle of inspiration.
    b. The highest airway resistance is in the smallest air conduits.
    c. The linear velocity of air flow falls progressively with each generation number of respiratory passages.
    d. Alveolar surface tension accounts for more than half the lung elastic recoil.
    e. The lungs exhibit much less hysteresis with respect to intra-alveolar pressure change than in the presence of a pneumothorax.

5.26 The pulmonary circulation differs from the systemic circulation in the following respects:

    a. Its peripheral vascular resistance is more evenly distributed between arterioles, capillaries and veins.
    b. It has a greater percentage of its blood volume in its capillaries than has the systemic circulation in the systemic capillaries.
    c. Its veins have no valves.
    d. The blood flow in its capillaries are pulsatile while those in the systemic circulation capillaries are not.
    e. Its capillaries undergo vasoconstriction with an acidosis.

5.27 In the case of pulmonary surfactant:

    a. The Clara cells of the respiratory bronchioles have a role in its production.
    b. Its protein components are synthesised in the Type II alveolar cells.
    c. Its production depends to a considerable extent on recycling of old surfactant.
    d. Its production in the near-term fetus is dependent on maternal glucocorticoids.
    e. It requires a mesh of tubular myelin spread on the alveolar epithelium for its proper function.

5.28 In the case of nitric oxide:

a. It is a free radical.
b. It is an autacoid.
c. It is synthesised in the brain.
d. It is a positive cardiac inotrope.
e. Its production is enhanced by glucocorticoids.

5.29 A rise in the plasma concentration of the following normally leads to vasodilatation:

a. Sodium.
b. Calcium.
c. Glucose.
d. Citrate.
e. Bradykinin.

5.30 The activity of warfarin is enhanced:

a. In old age.
b. During pregnancy.
c. By aspirin.
d. By barbiturates.
e. By metronidazole.

5.31 The following agents are inactivated on passage through the pulmonary circulation:

a. Arachidonic acid.
b. Antidiuretic hormone.
c. Bradykinin.
d. Dopamine.
e. 5-hydroxytryptamine.

5.32 Albumin:

a. Is a polydispersed colloid.
b. Is synthesised only in the liver.
c. Contains no carbohydrate moieties in its structure.
d. Exerts a higher osmotic pressure in the plasma than does globulin.
e. Usually falls in its plasma concentration after major surgery.

5.33 **Blood:**

    a. Is a newtonian fluid.
    b. Is a thixotropic fluid.
    c. Has a viscosity that has a direct linear relationship to its haematocrit.
    d. In the normal person has a viscosity about 1.5 times that of the plasma.
    e. In its passage through narrow conduits demonstrates the Fahraeus–Lindqvist phenomenon.

5.34 **The following are higher in the cerebrospinal fluid than in the plasma:**

    a. pH.
    b. Magnesium.
    c. Calcium.
    d. Urea.
    e. pCO_2.

5.35 **Concerning body temperature change under general anaesthesia:**

    a. The core temperature falls during the first hour predominantly from reduced heat production.
    b. In general the core skin temperature gradient increases.
    c. Conduction is the predominant mode of heat loss.
    d. Convection heat loss is increased by a 'wind chill' effect in the theatre environment.
    e. Increased humidity of theatre environment will tend to retard the fall in body temperature.

5.36 **Concerning the kidneys:**

    a. Together they weigh about the same as the heart.
    b. Their total oxygen consumption (ml/minute) is greater than that of the heart.
    c. They have a higher blood flow per unit mass compared with the liver.
    d. Their venous oxygen saturation is lower than that of the brain (jugular venous bulb O_2 saturation).
    e. They expend about the same percentage of their energy (determined as basal O_2 consumption) for sodium re-absorption as does the brain for maintaining the electrical gradient across its neuronal membranes.

Physics and equipment

5.37   The following are SI units:

a. Dyne.
b. Centimetre.
c. Siemens.
d. Stokes.
e. Farad.

5.38   The following pairs are exactly equal in magnitude:

a. 1 degree celsius and 1 kelvin.
b. 1 mmHg and 1 torr.
c. 1 litre and 1/1000 of a cubic metre.
d. 1 angstrom and 0.1 nanometre.
e. 1 mho and 1 siemens.

5.39   The units attached to each of the following physical quantities are correct:

a. Stress: newtons per square metre.
b. Surface tension: joules per square metre.
c. Resistance (to air flow in lungs): cm water pressure.
d. Magnetic flux: tesla.
e. Dynamic viscosity: pascals per second.

5.40   The following are 'dimensionless entities', i.e. they are mere numbers or ratios or percentages and have no units attached to them:

a. Fluoride number.
b. Cell wall permeability.
c. Substitution index.
d. Osmotic coefficient.
e. Avogadro's constant.

5.41   The following are graded according to steel wire gauge (SWG):

a. Tuohy needles.
b. Intravenous cannulae.
c. Epidural catheters.
d. Paediatric orotracheal tubes.
e. Nasogastric tubes.

5.42 **The piezo-electric principle:**

a. Is a principle that is operational in invasive arterial blood pressure monitoring.
b. Can be used for analysis of halogenated inhalational anaesthetic agents.
c. Is an essential application in ultrasound diagnostics.
d. Is a necessary pre-requisite in magnetic resonance imaging.
e. Is utilised in the measurement of temperature using a Bourdon gauge-type instrument.

5.43 **The following are by definition transducers:**

a. The retina of the human eye.
b. The fluid coupled diaphragm unit for invasive blood pressure measurement.
c. A mercury sphygmomanometer.
d. An AC step-down transformer.
e. The piezoelectric crystal in an ultrasound diagnostic machine.

5.44 **The following are attributes associated with diathermy (electrosurgery):**

a. Duty cycle.
b. Current density.
c. Interrogation current.
d. Channelling.
e. Crest factor.

5.45 **The accuracy of invasive arterial blood pressure monitoring is enhanced if the fluid-coupled catheter system incorporates the following features:**

a. A larger volume dome.
b. A stiffer diaphragm.
c. A stiff-walled catheter.
d. Long tubing.
e. Avoidance of air bubbles.

5.46 The following statements are true:

a. The amperage required to induce ventricular fibrillation is higher than that required to produce cardiac standstill.

b. The electrical impedance of an operating theatre floor must be of a higher degree so as to provide safety from electrocution than that required to render an anaesthetic machine free from static electricity.

c. The voltage required to make a DC defibrillator properly functional must be higher than the mains voltage.

d. The duration of an electric current for successful electroconvulsive therapy (ECT) is greater than that required for each TOF stimulation when using a PNS.

e. The active stage of diathermy current during its coagulation mode is longer than during its cutting mode.

5.47 The following are essential prerequisites for the functioning of a defibrillator for manual DC conversion of ventricular fibrillation:

a. A built-in transformer.

b. The presence of a rectifier in the circuit.

c. A capacitor.

d. An inductor.

e. A synchroniser unit.

5.48 The following devices measure temperature by detecting a change in electrical resistance:

a. Platinum resistance thermometer.

b. Thermistor.

c. Thermocouple.

d. Bimetallic strip thermometer.

e. Bourdon gauge thermometer.

5.49 The operational frequencies when using the following devices are in the range of about 10–50 Hz:

a. Resonant frequency of a fluid coupled system for invasive arterial BP measurement.

b. EEG machine.

c. Peripheral nerve stimulator when used for TOF stimulation.

d. Battery-operated portable defibrillator.

e. TENS machine.

5.50   The following are attributes of ultrasound:

   a. Cavitation.
   b. Acoustic mismatch.
   c. Precession.
   d. Collimation.
   e. Larmor frequency.

5.51   The following gases for medical and/or industrial use are
        obtained by fractional distillation of air:

   a. Oxygen.
   b. Nitrogen.
   c. Helium.
   d. Carbon dioxide.
   e. Xenon.

5.52   According to international convention the bodies of medical gas
        cylinders are colour coded as follows:

   a. Entonox: blue and white.
   b. Air: black.
   c. 5% CO_2 in oxygen: black.
   d. Cyclopropane: orange.
   e. Nitrogen: grey.

5.53   The following cylinders, no matter their size, have a gas
        pressure of about 137 bar when full:

   a. Carbon dioxide.
   b. 5% CO_2 in oxygen.
   c. Cyclopropane.
   d. Helium.
   e. Nitrogen.

5.54   Helium:

   a. Is an essential element for the working of the MRI scanner.
   b. Is an integral element in the performance of the CO_2 laser.
   c. Is an appropriate peritoneal insufflation gas at laparoscopy.
   d. Is a useful adjuvant gas to relieve the difficulty of oxygenation
      in bronchial asthma.
   e. Is a useful inhalational adjunct in deep sea diving.

5.55 **An adiabatic change:**

a. Is a physical change in a system unaccompanied by heat exchange between the system and the outside.
b. Is a condition that must prevail if Boyle's law is to hold good.
c. Is exemplified by the Joule–Thomson effect.
d. Must necessarily occur so as to obtain oxygen by the process of fractional distillation of air.
e. Can occur at the Bodok seal interface on the anaesthetic machine on opening a cylinder of oxygen.

5.56 **The following have been known to accumulate in low-flow breathing attachments as a reaction between inhalational anaesthetic agents and soda lime:**

a. Trifluoromethyl vinyl ether.
b. Dichloroacetylene.
c. Acetone.
d. Nitrogen dioxide.
e. Methane.

5.57 **The 'TEC Mark 6' Desflurane vaporiser:**

a. Is based on the 'copper kettle' principle.
b. Is calibrated using air.
c. Contains an in-built 'pressure-regulating' valve.
d. Has a 'working pressure' that has a direct linear relationship with the fresh gas flow rate.
e. Performs accurately, even at different altitudes.

5.58 **The following drugs on biotransformation produce metabolites that have the same main pharmacological action as the parent agent:**

a. Morphine.
b. Suxamethonium.
c. Midazolam.
d. Vecuronium.
e. Pethidine.

5.59 **The following anti-emetics mediate their action predominantly by acting at D_2 (dopamine 2) receptors:**

a. Promethazine.
b. Scopolamine.
c. Metoclopramide.
d. Ondansetron.
e. Dexamethasone.

5.60 **Aspirin:**

a. Is absorbed in the stomach by passive diffusion down a concentration gradient.
b. Is well bound to plasma globulin.
c. Undergoes extensive first-pass metabolism in the liver.
d. Has an effect on platelet function that cannot be measured by routine laboratory tests of coagulation.
e. Has a much longer pharmacodynamic half-life than a pharmacokinetic half-life.

5.61 **Aspirin:**

a. Suppresses leukotriene formation.
b. Inactivates cyclo-oxygenase by covalent modification of the enzyme.
c. Provides pain relief by a predominantly direct central action.
d. Is eliminable from the body by forced acid diuresis.
e. In excess causes permanent tinnitus.

5.62 **Metformin:**

a. Is a biguanide.
b. Is a hypoglycaemic agent.
c. Is absorbed mainly in the duodenum.
d. Binds avidly to plasma proteins.
e. Is excreted as a glucuronide in the urine.

5.63 **Elicitation of neuromuscular block using a peripheral nerve stimulator is more accurate and reliable:**

a. If the electrodes are placed nearest the muscle to be tested.
b. If the skin surface for electrodes is cooler rather than warmer.
c. When tactile rather than visual method of evaluation of response is employed.
d. When using the ulnar nerve, response of the thumb rather than the little finger is observed.
e. If supramaximal rather than submaximal stimulation is used.

5.64 **The following statements are true with respect to neuromuscular stimulation:**

a. Absence of 'fade' in TOF mode excludes the presence of residual NM blockade.
b. 'Fade' in response to tetanic stimulation is regarded as a postsynaptic event.
c. Phase II block is also known as 'dual block'.
d. Post-tetanic potentiation is characteristic of partial non-depolarisation block.
e. Return of muscle power of the adductor pollicis muscle usually means return of diaphragmatic activity.

5.65 The following impair neuromuscular transmission at skeletal muscle NM junctions by decreasing acetylcholine release at the pre-synaptic site:

a. Verapamil.
b. Steroids.
c. Tetracyclines.
d. Magnesium.
e. Furosemide.

5.66 Non-depolarising NMBAs differ from depolarising NMBAs in the following respects:

a. The former are antagonists at the NMJ, the latter are partial agonists.
b. The former act competitively, the latter non-competitively.
c. The former need to bind to just one α subunit of the receptor to effect their action, the latter need to bind to both.
d. The former show 'fade' on TOF stimulation, the latter do not.
e. The former show a more pronounced action in the Eaton–Lambert syndrome, the latter do not.

5.67 In the case of thiopentone sodium:

a. It is marketed as a racemic mixture.
b. Its solubility is sharply increased on injection into the bloodstream.
c. It owes its action to its ability to assume the ketotautomeric form in vivo.
d. It contains disodium edetate as a bacterial retardant.
e. It contains sodium bicarbonate to maintain its alkalinity.

5.68 The following anaesthetic agents bring about their effects by acting at GABA receptors:

a. Thiopentone.
b. Methohexitone.
c. Propofol.
d. Etomidate.
e. Ketamine.

5.69 Thiopentone solution is not compatible with the following, forming a precipitate with them on mixing:

a. Vecuronium.
b. Pethidine.
c. Atracurium.
d. Suxamethonium.
e. Hartmann's solution.

5.70 Recovery from the pharmacological effects of the following are essentially by redistribution of the agents:

a. Thiopentone sodium.
b. Propofol.
c. Halothane.
d. Benzodiazepines.
e. Ketamine.

5.71 The following are additives found in benzodiazepine preparations:

a. Propylene glycol.
b. Cremophor EL.
c. Sodium benzoate.
d. Hydrochloric acid.
e. Sodium carbonate.

5.72 Each of the following is lower for desflurane compared with the other halogenated inhalational agents: halothane, enflurane, isoflurane and sevoflurane:

a. MAC.
b. Boiling point.
c. Blood-gas partition coefficient.
d. Biotransformation.
e. Tendency to form carbon monoxide with soda lime.

5.73 Of the currently used local anaesthetic agents:

a. Cocaine is the only naturally occurring agent.
b. Prilocaine is the only one that causes methaemoglobinaemia.
c. Ropivacaine is the only synthetic LA with vasoconstrictor activity.
d. Lignocaine is the only achiral agent.
e. Bupivacaine is the only one that is available as a pure enantiomer.

5.74 Morphine differs from fentanyl and its congeners in the following respects:

a. It shows no 'ceiling effect' with regard to respiratory depression.
b. There is little transient first-pass uptake by the lungs.
c. It has a lower percentage of bound to plasma proteins.
d. It produces glucuronides on Phase II biotransformation.
e. It has no tendency to produce muscle rigidity.

5.75 The following are pure opioid antagonists:

a. Nalorphine.
b. Levallorphan.
c. Naloxone.
d. Naltrexone.
e. Buprenorphine.

5.76 Codeine:

a. Is structurally a phenanthrene.
b. Is a pro-drug.
c. Has a better oral–parenteral potency ratio than morphine.
d. Is a poorer antitussive than morphine.
e. Causes more constipation than morphine.

5.77 The following antiemetics produce their effects by acting on the chemoreceptor trigger zone (CTZ) rather than on the vomiting centre itself:

a. Cyclizine.
b. Antimuscarinics.
c. Corticosteroids.
d. Droperidol.
e. Metoclopramide.

5.78 The following reduce gastric acidity by a process of pharmacological antagonism:

a. Sodium citrate.
b. Magnesium trisilicate.
c. Carbenoxolone.
d. Ranitidine.
e. Omeprazole.

5.79 The speed of induction of an inhalational anaesthetic agent is directly proportional to:

a. The blood-gas partition coefficient of the agent.
b. The MAC of the agent.
c. Alveolar ventilation.
d. Cardiac output.
e. Percentage of adipose tissue in the body.

5.80 **In myasthenia gravis:**

a. The disease when appearing in males occurs later in life than in females.
b. The weakness is in the distal muscles rather than the proximal muscles.
c. The muscle weakness is worse at the start of the day than toward the end of the day.
d. Thymectomy can lead to improvement even in the absence of a thymoma.
e. Progressive wasting of muscles is a common manifestation.

5.81 **Concerning acute porphyria:**

a. It has a sex-linked autosomal dominant inheritance.
b. It is more common in men than in women.
c. Its highest incidence is in the third and fourth decades of life.
d. Enzyme-inducing drugs are more likely to precipitate the condition than non-enzyme-inducing agents.
e. Cimetidine is an effective prophylactic against attacks.

5.82 **In the case of obstructive sleep apnoea:**

a. It is estimated to be present in about 50% of obese persons.
b. It usually occurs in early youth.
c. It is more common in women than in men.
d. Its mechanism of production is a decrease in pharyngeal muscle tone during sleep.
e. It is associated with mid-afternoon headaches.

5.83 **Concerning malignant hyperpyrexia:**

a. It has a strict autosomal dominant inheritance.
b. It has a higher incidence in adults than in children.
c. Where death occurs inhalational anaesthetic agents are invariably implicated.
d. The earliest sign of its presence is invariably a rising temperature.
e. The acid-base derangement that accompanies it is a respiratory acidosis with a compensatory metabolic alkalosis.

5.84 **Magnesium:**

a. Is absorbed by an active process in the duodenum.
b. Is carried in the plasma unbound.
c. Is an essential co-factor of Na^+–K^+–ATPase.
d. Is an integral element of NMDA channels.
e. Is essential for end-organ response to parathyroid hormone.

5.85 Administration of 8.4% sodium bicarbonate to correct a metabolic acidosis can lead to:

a. Plasma hyperosmolarity.
b. Hypernatraemia.
c. Hypokalaemia.
d. A raised haemoglobin P_{50}.
e. Intracellular acidosis.

5.86 The following processes are necessarily enzyme dependent:

a. Conversion of CO_2 to $-HCO_3$ within the red cell.
b. Breakdown of suxamethonium in the plasma.
c. Production of nitric oxide.
d. Biotransformation of atracurium.
e. Conversion of arachidonic acid to prostaglandins.

5.87 Concerning isomerism:

a. Enflurane and isoflurane are stereo-isomers of each other.
b. Geometric isomerism is a form of stereo-isomerism.
c. Keto-enol isomerism is one form of lactam-lactim isomerism.
d. *Cis-trans* isomerism is only possible in compounds containing carbon–carbon double bonds.
e. Achiral compounds are not capable of existence as racemates.

5.88 Of the interatomic attractions and bonds: ionic bonds, covalent bonds, hydrogen bonds, van der Waals' attractions and London forces:

a. Ionic bonds are energetically the strongest.
b. Covalent bonding is the norm in antagonist–receptor unions that lead to irreversible pharmacological inhibition.
c. Hydrogen bonding is only present in water.
d. Van der Waals' attractions in gas molecules are responsible for the 'ideal' behaviour of gases.
e. London forces are only possible in molecules of polar compounds.

5.89 The following pairs refer to the same thing:

a. Joule–Thomson effect and Joule–Kelvin effect.
b. Dielectric constant and relative permittivity.
c. Amphotericity and amphipathicity.
d. Mho and siemens.
e. Channel-mediated diffusion and facilitated diffusion.

5.90 The following statements are true:

a. All materials are diamagnetic by nature.
b. All bodies emit electromagnetic radiations.
c. All gases necessarily become solids at temperatures near 0 K.
d. All amino acids in the body containing asymmetrical carbon atoms are *l*-amino acids.
e. All sugars need to be converted into monosaccharides to be capable of absorption in the intestine.

5.1 Answers

a. True.

b. False – the 2nd thoracic nerve also contributes, not through the brachial plexus, but by an independent intercostobrachial nerve that crosses the axilla to reach the arm.

c. False – the trapezius muscle is supplied by the spinal part of the accessory nerve and the ventral rami of C3 and C4.

d. False – the posterior cord does.

e. False – the serratus anterior is supplied by the long thoracic nerve (of Bell), which arises directly from the *roots* of C3, C4 and C5.

5.2 Answers

a. True – the cranial parasympathetic outflow is via cranial nerves III, VII, X and XI.

b. False – enters the orbit as two branches, upper and lower.

c. False – except the lateral rectus and superior oblique muscles.

d. True – the parasympathetic outflow via the ciliary ganglion to the sphincter pupillae muscle.

e. True – the parasympathetic (constrictor) supply to the pupil (see d.)

5.3 Answers

a. True.

b. True.

c. False.

d. False.

e. True.

Note: A 'tight junction' (or *zona occludens*) is a structure that impedes the passage of molecules and ions *between* cells and consists of parallel strands of closely packed particles, and the degree of 'tightness' of the junction is related to the number of these parallel strands. They are: (i) barriers, which completely block the flow of ions and water between cells; (ii) selective gates, which permit certain solutes to flow more easily than others; and (iii) fences, which separate the polarised surfaces of the epithelial membrane into apical and basolateral domains.

5.4 Answers

a. False – T10 provides the cutaneous supply to the abdominal wall at the level of the umbilicus.

b. False.

c. False.

d. True – L1: iliohypogastric, ilio-inguinal and genitofemoral nerves.

e. True. L2: genitofemoral nerve.

5.5 Answers

a. **True**.
b. **True**.
c. **True**.
d. **False** – the lumbar vertebrae also increase in size progressively from up downwards.
e. **True**.

5.6 Answers

a. **False** – it increases.
b. **True**.
c. **False** – the dicrotic notch is attenuated.
d. **False** – pressure pulse wave velocity: 3–14 ms^{-1}, 15–100 times faster than the rate of blood flow.
e. **True**.

5.7 Answers

a. **True**. c. 60–70 ml of a ventricular end-diastolic volume of 100–120 ml.
b. **False** – the energy for cardiac muscle contraction is derived mainly from oxidative metabolism of fatty acids and to a lesser extent from glucose.
c. **False** – only about 20–25%; the rest of the (chemical) energy is converted to heat.
d. **True**.
e. **False** – as the heart rate increases, both systole and diastole shorten, but the diastolic phase shortens more than the systolic phase. Therefore the ratio increases.

5.8 Answers

a. **True** – because the excitation wave starts in the sinoatrial node, which is sited in the right atrium.
b. **True** – it is for this reason that the right atrium is taken as the reference point for both central venous and arterial blood pressure measurements.
c. **True**.
d. **True** – Bainbridge reflex: stretching of low-pressure atrial receptors, as a result of increased filling of the right atrium, leads to a reflex tachycardia.
e. **False** – although the right atrium is the predominant site of ANP release, all four cardiac chambers are regarded as sites of production of the hormone.

5.9 Answers

a. True – Bezold–Jarisch reflex: the response, by way of the triad of bradycardia, hypotension and coronary dilatation, to stimuli sensed by chemo- and mechano-receptors within the ventricular wall.

b. True – increased stretch of the ventricular muscle fibres will lead to more forceful contraction of the ventricular musculature. In other words, 'the energy of contraction is a function of the ventricular muscle fibre length'.

c. False – Stress–relaxation: ability of smooth muscle to return nearly to its original force of contraction seconds or minutes after it has been elongated or shortened. A phenomenon particularly of blood vessels, it is not an attribute of the ventricular musculature because the ventricle is a 'rapid response' organ to changes in blood pressure or intraventricular blood volume.

d. False – Latch bridge mechanism: sustained contraction of smooth muscle for some time after removal of stimulus and resulting from myosin cross-bridges remaining attached to actin for some time after fall in cytoplasmic Ca^{2+} concentrations. It is not a phenomenon of cardiac muscle, whose responses are 'phasic', contraction alternating with relaxation. In vascular smooth muscle contraction must necessarily be 'tonic'.

e. False – Paul Bert effect: central nervous system damage from oxygen toxicity. It has nothing to do with cardiac activity.

5.10 Answers

a. False – in the AV node. Velocity of conduction in atrial muscle: $1.0–1.2$ ms^{-1}; AV node: $0.02–0.1$ ms^{-1}; Bundle of His: $1.2–2.0$ ms^{-1}; Purkinje fibres: $2.0–4.0$ ms^{-1}.

b. True.

c. True.

d. True – a rate of c. 20/minute.

e. True – neither has the atrial musculature.

5.11 Answers

a. True – about two-thirds of the vascular resistance resides in the arterioles.

b. False – more than 50% of the blood volume is in the venous compartment, about 15–20% in the pulmonary circulation, and only about 30–35% is on the arterial side: heart: c. 300–400 ml; aorta: c. 400–500 ml; arteries: c. 500–600 ml; arterioles: c. 50–100 ml; capillaries: c. 250 ml.

c. False – the relationship is inverse.

d. True.

e. False – the relationship is direct, but not linear. The COP increases disproportionately with increase in plasma protein concentration because of the Gibbs–Donnan effect.

5.12 Answers

a. **False** – in all pressure measurements in the circulatory system the zero reference point is the right atrium. Therefore the mercury zero too ought to be at that level.
b. **False** – it will give a lower value.
c. **False** – the greater the reading error.
d. **False** – it is less correct because of the pressure drop along the tube during cuff deflation.
e. **False** – the cuff width ought to be about 20% longer than the arm diameter.

5.13 Answers

a. **True** – it contains one haem moiety combined with one globin chain, compared with haemoglobin, which has four haem moieties, each combined with a globin chain, alpha or beta. The whole structure, four haems and two pairs of alpha and beta globin chains is haemoglobin.
b. **True** – cytochrome oxidase is a haemoprotein and is the terminal component of the mitochondrial respiratory carrier chain responsible for electron transfer to oxygen, the electrons having been released by the activity of dehydrogenases.
c. **False** – bilirubin is a linear tetrapyrrole.
d. **False** – protoporphyrin has no Fe^{2+}. The presence of iron is an essential pre-requisite for porphyrins to be labelled 'haem'.
e. **True** – but only in respect of soluble (i.e. cytosolic) guanylyl cyclase, which is the receptor protein for nitric oxide activity. This soluble guanylyl cyclase is totally unrelated to the receptor guanylyl cyclase responsible for the activity of cell surface G protein-coupled receptors.

5.14 Answers

a. **False** – it is a monomer because it has only one haem moiety and one globin chain per molecule.
b. **False** – myoglobin acts as an oxygen store, not an oxygen transporter.
c. **False** – its P_{50} is c. 5 mmHg (0.67 kPa); for HbF: c. 20 mmHg (2.67 kPa); for HbA: c. 27 mmHg (3.67 kPa).
d. **True**.
e. **False** – because the distal histidine in myoglobin causes 'steric hindrance' to CO bonding with myoglobin. Nevertheless, a small amount (c. 1%) of myoglobin is normally present in the body as myoglobin-CO.

5.15 Answers

a. False.

b. True.

c. True – although it is not an enzyme-activated process, the combination behaves as it were allosterically driven, i.e. the more oxygen combined with haemoglobin, the greater the affinity of haemoglobin for oxygen. In other words 'its appetite grows with eating'!

d. False – one molecule of oxygen combines with each of the four haem moieties of the haemoglobin molecule. Therefore 4 O_2 molecules combine with one haemoglobin molecule.

e. True.

5.16 Answers

a. False.

b. False – the reaction between CO_2 and H_2O inside red cells is catalysed by carbonic anhydrase and therefore is several 1000 times faster than without the enzyme; it is also faster than the combination of CO_2 with haemoglobin.

c. False – CO_2 combines with the amino groups of the globin chains.

d. False – the globin chains move further apart.

e. False – leads to the Bohr effect. The Haldane effect occurs when CO_2 is unloaded in the lungs.

5.17 Answers

a. True.

b. False.

c. True.

d. False.

e. False.

5.18 Answers

a. True – hence the role of aspirin as an anti-inflammatory agent by blocking cyclo-oxygenase.

b. True – prostaglandins are vasoactive and cause a change in vessel calibre, and are particularly important in regulation of renal blood flow.

c. True – by regulating the activity of the $Na^+–K^+–ATPase$ pump.

d. True.

e. True.

5.19 Answers

a. **True**.

b. **False** – ephedrine is *not* a catecholamine. It does not have two OH groups on its phenol moiety, therefore it is broken down neither by MAO nor COMT. It is excreted virtually unchanged in the urine.

c. **False** – acetylcholine is catalysed by acetylcholinesterase.

d. **True** – serotonin is metabolised primarily by type A MAO (which also breaks down noradrenaline) although it also has additional alternative routes of inactivation.

e. **False** – histamine is broken down by diamine oxidase. MAO does metabolise its breakdown products methylhistamine and methylimidazole acetic acid, but not histamine itself.

5.20 Answers

a. **False** – it is a nonapeptide.

b. **True** – vasopressin and oxytocin differ in respect of only two out of their nine amino acids: phenylalanine and arginine in the former and isoleucine and leucine in the latter. For this reason each of them has some of the activity of the other: c. 10–20%.

c. **True**.

d. **True** – ADH promotes the release of ACTH from the anterior pituitary by an action on V_3 receptors (previously known as V_{1B} receptors).

e. **False** – V_2 receptors.

Note: vasopressin receptors are of three types: V_{1A}, V_{1B} and V_2. V_{1A} receptors are those responsible for mediating the blood pressure effects, V_{1B} for ACTH release from anterior pituitary (see **d**), and V_2 for antidiuretic action.

5.21 Answers

a. **False** – it is the absence of brown fat that is a major factor in obesity.

b. **True** – thermogenin is the protein that is responsible for heat production.

c. **False** – it produces less ATP and therefore less free energy that is convertible into fat.

d. **True** – it is this that, again, leads to less fat accumulation.

e. **False** – it is the continuous dissipation of the proton gradient by thermogenin, which acts as a proton conductance pathway, through the membrane that causes heat release.

Note: Normally, the activity of the cellular respiratory chain produces heat in addition to translocating protons. The protons generate ATP when returning via F_1 ATP synthase and this ATP generation in mitochondria is therefore dependent on the inner mitochondrial membrane being impermeable to protons, thus forcing the protons to enter the mitochondrial matrix only via the ATP-generating channels.

In brown fat thermogenin acts as a proton conductance pathway through the membrane – a 'hole in the wall' – which in effect acts as a shortcut, bypassing the ATP generation pathway, thereby allowing a greater dissipation of heat than would otherwise happen in its absence.

5.22 Answers

a. **True**.

b. **True**.

c. **True**.

d. **False**.

e. **False**.

5.23 Answers

a. **False** – it is a 21-residue polypeptide.

b. **False** – it is a vasoconstrictor, one of the most potent of endogenous vasoconstrictors.

c. **True**.

d. **True**.

e. **True** – its vasoconstrictor effect is antagonised by NO.

5.24 Answers

a. True – because of: (i) loss of water into the interstitial space; and (ii) increase in size of red cells (see **c** below).

b. True – because of the acidity produced by CO_2, the pH drops from c. 7.4 to c. 7.36.

c. True – because of the formation of bicarbonate and therefore leading to an increase in the number of osmotically active particles, which then draw water into the red cells, making the cells about 0.5 μ larger in diameter.

d. True – formation of bicarbonate from CO_2 inside red cells under the influence of carbonic anhydrase leads to movement of $-HCO_3$ into the plasma down a concentration gradient. This leads to transfer of an equimolar amount of chloride into the red cell so as to maintain electroneutrality, thus leading to a slightly lower plasma chloride concentration in venous blood compared with arterial blood.

e. False – it is lower: the total pressure of dissolved gases in arterial blood is as follows: pO_2 c. 14 kPa; pN_2 c. 80 kPa; pCO_2 5.3 = c. 99.3. In venous blood the respective figures are: 5.3, 80 and 6.1 = 91.4 kPa.

5.25 Answers

a. False – the external intercostal muscles also have a role.

b. False – the highest resistance is in the pharynx and larynx and upper airways and lowest in the small airways: total airway resistance: 1.5 cm H_2O water per litre per second, 0.6 in the upper airways and only c. 0.3 in the lower airways.

c. False – in airway generation 2–4 the linear velocity rises c. 25–30% of that of generation 1 and only progressively declines after that to near zero in the alveoli.

d. True.

e. True.

5.26 Answers

a. True – about 30–40% each in the arteries, capillaries and the veins, compared with the systemic circulation, where 80% of the resistance is in the arterioles.

b. True – in the systemic circulation, c. 250 ml out of c. 4000 ml are in the capillaries. In the pulmonary circulation, it is c. 150–200 ml out of c. 800–1000 ml.

c. True.

d. True.

e. True – systemic capillaries dilate under acidotic conditions.

5.27 Answers

a. **True** – some of the components of surfactant are manufactured by Clara cells.

b. **True** – the four apoproteins, SP-A, -B, -C and -D, are synthesised in Type II cells.

c. **True** – two mechanisms are responsible for the fate of surfactant: (i) breakdown and removal by alveolar macrophages; and (ii) re-uptake by Type II cells, which then destroy it or recycle it.

d. **True** – near term there is a surge of glucocorticoid release into the maternal circulation, which causes a marked increase in surfactant production in the normal fetus.

e. **False** – when released into the water layer of the alveolar epithelium, surfactant takes the form of a mesh known as tubular myelin, which is rich in surfactant apoproteins. However, this transformation is not essential for surfactant activity because knockout mice lack the myelin network and yet have a normally functional alveolar surface film of surfactant.

Note: pulmonary surfactant is a mixture of dipalmitoylphosphatidylcholine (c.50%), phosphatidylcholine (c. 40%) and proteins (c.10%), of which half are plasma proteins (albumin and IgA) and the other half apoproteins. The proteins confer an immune function on surfactant by acting as bacteria-coating opsonins.

5.28 Answers

a. **True** – free radicals are metabolite intermediates containing a single unpaired electron in the outer orbital shells of their molecules: e.g. ROO' , RO', OH'. (oxygen has two unpaired electrons and therefore is a 'diradical').

b. **True** – autacoids are 'local hormones', i.e. they are released by cells and act on the same or very nearby cells.

c. **True**.

d. **False** – a negative cardiac inotrope.

e. **False** – glucocorticoids inhibit the expression of NO synthase and therefore the production of NO.

5.29 Answers

a. **True** – mild arteriolar dilatation from water attraction into the plasma compartment as a result of increased osmolarity.

b. **True**.

c. **True** – a higher glucose level leads to an increase in osmolarity, which draws water into the plasma compartment leading to vasodilatation to accommodate the extra water.

d. **True**.

e. **True** – bradykinin is an arteriolar vasodilator.

5.30 Answers

a. **True** – because of gradual diminution of the levels of clotting factors.
b. **False** – vitamin K-dependent coagulation factors are raised in pregnancy.
c. **True** – because of aspirin's action on platelet adhesiveness and therefore on haemostasis.
d. **False** – enzyme induction by barbiturates will lead to more rapid metabolism of warfarin.
e. **True** – because metronidazole displaces warfarin from its protein-bound sites.

5.31 Answers

a. **False** – arachidonic acid is activated to prostaglandins.
b. **False**.
c. **True** – 80% of bradykinin is inactivated during passage through the pulmonary circulation.
d. **False** – dopamine is not inactivated in its passage through the pulmonary circulation.
e. **True** – 98% is removed in a single pass.

5.32 Answers

a. **False** – albumin is a uniform protein and therefore is a monodispersed colloid compared with (say) the gelatin colloids, which are of different molecular weights and therefore are 'polydispersed' colloids.
b. **True**.
c. **True** – contrast globulins, which may be 'glycated'.
d. **True** – because its molecular weight (69,000) is lower than that of the globulins (average MW c. 140,000) and it is found in a higher concentration in the plasma: c. 45 g/L to globulins' c. 25 g/L. The osmotic pressure of albumin is c. 22 mmHg, globulins c.6 mmHg.
e. **True** – usually falls after major surgery, leading to a diminution in its osmotic pressure to c. 15 mmHg after 24 hours. The fall is partly at least due to water retention as a stress response to surgery.

5.33 Answers

a. **False** – a newtonian fluid is one in which the velocity gradient is directly proportional to the shear stress and thus behaves in conformity with the Hagen–Poiseuille (H–P) law, i.e. its flow is laminar and the flow rate is in accordance with the H–P equation. Blood is a non-newtonian fluid, i.e. its flow is non-laminar and therefore its flow rate cannot be determined by application of the H–P equation.

b. **True** – a thixotropic fluid is one whose viscosity varies with its velocity gradient, i.e. the flow rate and also the time for which it is applied. A thixotropic fluid becomes fluid when subjected to an applied stress. *Thixis* is Greek, meaning 'touching', and *trope* is Greek, meaning 'turning'.

c. **False** – the viscosity varies with haematocrit in the form of an accelerating growth exponential.

d. **False** – plasma has a viscosity c. 1.5 times that of water and blood with a haemoglobin of 15/dl. It has a viscosity c. 2.5 times that of plasma.

e. **True** – Fahraeus-Lindqvist phenomenon: the exhibition of a far lower viscosity of blood when it traverses minute blood vessels than larger blood vessels. It is caused by alignment of red cells in an orderly manner, thus minimising the viscous resistance that occurs internally in the blood itself.

5.34 Answers

a. **False** – it is marginally lower: CSF: 7.33; plasma: 7.40.
b. **True** – CSF: 1.1 mmol/L; plasma: 0.8 mmol/L
c. **False** – CSF: 1.2 mmol/L; plasma: 2.4 mmol/L.
d. **False** – the same: 2.5–7.5 mmol/L.
e. **True** – CSF: c. 7 kPa; plasma: c. 5.3 kPa.

5.35 Answers

a. **False** – the fall in the first hour is due to vasodilatation and transfer of heat from core to periphery.

b. **False** – it decreases for the reason given in **a**.

c. **False** – conduction accounts for only about 1–2% of heat loss from the human body, whether in the awake or anaesthetised person. The relative percentages of body heat loss in the normal person are: radiation: c. 40%; convection: c. 30%; respiration: 20%; perspiration: c.10%. Conduction only accounts for about 1–2% of normal loss of body heat. In the patient under general anaesthesia, especially with an open abdomen, evaporation accounts for a significantly greater percentage of heat loss.

d. **True** – theatre plenum ventilation produces a 'wind chill' effect on the body, leading to a fall in temperature.

e. **True** – evaporation, whether through perspiration or respiration, is the only means whereby a person can lose body heat against a temperature gradient, but it is contingent on the ambient air being relatively dry. Increased humidity of the air will make it more difficult to lose heat by this method and it is the cause of 'heat stroke' in a hot and humid environment.

5.36 Answers

a. **True** – about 300 g.

b. **False** – heart: c. 26 ml/minute, i.e. c. 10% of basal O_2 consumption; kidneys: c. 8%, i.e. c. 20 ml/minute.

c. **True** – liver: blood flow (hepatic artery + portal vein): c. 1400 ml/minute; weight: c. 1400 g. Therefore blood flow = c. 100 ml/100 g. Kidneys: blood flow c.1200 ml/minute; weight: 300 g. Therefore blood flow = c. 400 ml/100 g.

d. **False** – cerebral O_2 consumption: c. 50 ml/minute; cerebral blood flow: c. 700 ml/minute. Therefore O_2 extraction = c. 7 ml from every 100 ml blood. Therefore the venous O_2 content is 20–7, i.e. c. 13 ml. Renal blood flow: 1200 ml/minute; O_2 consumption: c. 20 ml/minute. Therefore oxygen extraction is 20/12 ml per 100 ml blood flow, i.e. 1.6 ml per 100 ml of blood. Therefore the renal vein O_2 content is > 18 ml per 100 ml blood. Note: for the purpose of the calculation the Hb is assumed to be 15 g/dl of blood.

e. **True** – c. 60–65% for maintaining the Na^+–K^+–ATPase pump for either purpose.

5.37 Answers

a. False – the dyne is the unit of force in the CGS system. The corresponding SI unit is the newton.

b. False – the corresponding SI unit is 10×10^{-3} of a metre.

c. True – it is the unit of electrical conductance. The former unit was the mho, i.e. the reciprocal of the ohm. Note: the expression is '1 siemens', i.e. the form is plural, because it is named after Ernst Werner von Siemens (1816–1892).

d. False – it is the CGS unit of kinematic viscosity that is equal to the ratio of the dynamic viscosity (in poise) to the density (in grams per cubic centimetres). Note, again, the plural form '1 stokes' because it is named after Sir George Stokes.

e. True – it is the SI unit of electrical capacitance.

5.38 Answers

a. True.

b. False – there is a difference of c. 2 parts in 10 million between them.

c. False – 1 L is 'the volume of 1 kg of pure water at 4°C at standard pressure', which is equal to $1.000\ 028\ dm^3$, which is fractionally more than $1/1000$ of a m^3.

d. True – 1 Å = 10^{-10} m; 1 nm = 10^{-9} m.

e. True – the siemens replaced the mho as the unit of electrical conductance in the SI convention (reciprocal of resistance, the unit of which is the ohm). See answers to question **6.37**.

5.39 Answers

a. True – stress is the same as force per unit area, i.e. pressure.

b. True – surface tension is normally expressed as 'newtons per metre', which is the same as 'joules per square metre'.

c. False – cm water per litres gas flow per second.

d. False – magnetic flux: weber. Magnetic flux density: tesla. Magnetic flux density is magnetic flux per unit area, i.e. webers per m^2.

e. False – newton seconds per m^2 or pascal seconds.

5.40 Answers

a. **True** – the percentage inhibition of cholinesterase by 5×10^{-5} molar sodium fluoride.

b. **False** – net rate of diffusion of a substance for a unit area of the membrane for a unit concentration gradient between the two sides of the membrane.

c. **True** – the average number of hydroxyethyl groups per glucose moiety in hydroxyethyl starch preparations.

d. **True** – the degree to which an electrolyte (e.g. NaCl) is dissociated. If the dissociation is 100%, then the coefficient is 1.0; if it is less than 100%, then it is proportionately less than 1.0.

e. **False** – Avogadro's constant: number of molecules in 1 gmol of a gas at STP, which is 6.02×10^{23} per mole. Therefore the units are: $mole^{-1}$.

5.41 Answers

a. **True**.

b. **True**.

c. **True**.

d. **False** – orotracheal tubes are gauged according to their internal and external diameters in millimetres.

e. **False** – graded according to French catheter gauge (FCG).

Note: FCG is a unit with dimensions. It is the external circumference of the device in millimetres. SWG has no dimensions; it refers to the number of the particular device that can be accommodated in a standard measuring device. For this reason the higher the SWG number, the smaller the bore of the device, for example cannulae.

5.42 Answers

a. **True** – the transducer of an invasive arterial BP measuring device converts a pressure signal into an electric signal, i.e. it is a piezo-electric device.

b. **True** – it is based on the principle that a piezo-electric crystal vibrates at a specific resonant frequency when energised by electricity. When coated with a lipid that adsorbs inhalational anaesthetics, the resonant frequency of the crystal decreases in proportion to the degree of adsorption of the agent, which in turn depends on the concentration of the anaesthetic agent.

c. **True** – the piezo-electric crystal of the ultrasound probe converts an electric current into an ultrasound wave, and vice versa.

d. **False**.

e. **False** – the change here is of heat into pressure change of a gas.

5.43 Answers

a. True – converts light energy into electrical energy.
b. True – converts mechanical energy into electrical energy.
c. False – there is no conversion of one type of energy into another; it is all mechanical energy.
d. False – a transformer merely changes the voltage of AC electricity.
e. True – as the name suggests, a 'piezo-electric' device converts pressure energy into electrical energy. In ultrasound the piezo-crystal converts energy from electricity to sound energy and vice versa.

Note: a transducer is a device that converts one form of energy into another.

5.44 Answers

a. True – the ratio of the time for which a unit is activated to the total duration of the on–off cycle of a periodically repeated operation. In cutting mode the duty cycle is 100%; in coagulation mode it is about 5–10%.
b. True – current density = watts per unit surface area of application. It is necessarily very high at the point of application of the diathermy probe and must necessarily be maintained very low under the diathermy plate so as to prevent a diathermy skin burn under the plate.
c. True – a physiologically benign current (of c. 2 mA and frequency of c. 140 kHz) that 'interrogates', i.e. checks the adequacy of contact between the diathermy plate and skin and sounds a warning if it falls below a critical level. It is a method for preventing skin burns under the diathermy plate.
d. True – the passage of the diathermy current along a pathway (especially an attenuated pathway) other than the intended pathway, thus leading to tissue heating and damage.
e. True – the ratio of the peak voltage to the root mean square (RMS) voltage of the diathermy current. The crest factor is higher (c.3.0) for coagulation mode compared with cutting mode (c.1.4) because the duty cycle (see **a**) is only about 5% for coagulating current compared with near 100% for cutting current.

5.45 Answers

a. False – a larger volume dome will increase the damping.
b. True – a stiff diaphragm will reduce the damping.
c. True – this will reduce the damping.
d. False – this will increase the damping.
e. True – this will reduce the damping.

5.46 Answers

a. **False** – VF: c. 80–100 mA; cardiac standstill: of the order of amperes.
b. **True**.
c. **True** – mains voltage (AC): 240 V RMS. DC defibrillator: c. 5000 V.
d. **True** – ECT current duration: 1–3 ms; PNS current duration: c. 200 μs.
e. **False** – 'duty cycle': coagulation mode: c. 5% of the total possible time of current application. For cutting mode it is 100% of the time of current application (see **6.44 a**.)

5.47 Answers

a. **True** – because the mains voltage of 240 V must be stepped up to about 5000 V. Note: this must be done before converting the AC electricity to DC.
b. **True** – the purpose of a rectifier (also called a 'diode') is to convert AC electricity to DC electricity.
c. **True** – necessary to store the electric charge and have it available for delivery to the patient.
d. **False** – an inductor is not absolutely necessary, but its presence helps to render the electric discharge pulse of optimum shape and duration so as to improve the effectiveness of defibrillation.
e. **False** – a synchroniser is not essential in a defibrillator that is used merely for correction of ventricular fibrillation. However, since defibrillators are used for synchronised DC cardioconversion as well, all present-day defibrillators are equipped with synchroniser units.

5.48 Answers

a. **True** – as its name implies it is a 'resistance' thermometer.
b. **True** – it measures the change in electrical resistance of a semi-conductor.
c. **False** – it measures the potential difference created between two junctions of two dissimilar metals.
d. **False** – it measures the degree of 'unfurling' of the strip as a result of the differential change in lengths of two strips of metal.
e. **False** – it measures the degree of 'unfurling' of a hollow coiled tube as a result of pressure change resulting from a change in temperature.

5.49 Answers

a. **True**.
b. **True** – about 25–30 Hz.
c. **False** – 2 Hz.
d. **False** – defibrillators are now 'DC'. The fact that they can be battery operated and portable is a red herring.
e. **False** – can be up to 200 Hz.

5.50 Answers

a. **True** – the high frequency waves can cause a high peak pressure in tissues, leading to the formation of microbubbles in tissue fluid. If these were to expand they could do so to the point of very sudden collapse and this will lead to 'cavitation'. There could also be a huge rise in temperature, leading to damage to cells.

b. **True** – where there is a media interface during ultrasound transmission, if the two media have markedly different acoustic impedances, then there is bound to be acoustic mismatch. The practical result of this is that a greater percentage of sound waves will be reflected at the interface compared with those that are transmitted.

c. **False** – precession is a property of MRI.

d. **False** – collimation (or non-divergence of light beam) is a property of laser light.

e. **False** – Larmor frequency applies to MRI.

5.51 Answers

a. **True**.

b. **True**.

c. **False** – helium is obtained from natural gas.

d. **False** – in the UK CO_2 is manufactured by three means: (i) as a by-product gas from manufacture of hydrogen; (ii) as a by-product gas from fermentation; and (iii) as a combustion gas from burning fuel.

e. **True**.

5.52 Answers

a. **False** – body: blue; shoulder: alternating blue and white.

b. **False** – body: grey; shoulder: alternating black and white.

c. **True** – body: black; shoulder: alternating white and grey.

d. **True** – both body and shoulder are orange.

e. **False** – body: black; shoulder: grey.

5.53 Answers

a. **False** – about 50 bar.

b. **True**.

c. **False** – about 7 bar.

d. **True**.

e. **True**.

5.54 Answers

a. **True** – it helps to supercool the electric coils to near 0 K and thereby render the cables superconducting.

b. **True** – it helps maintain 'population inversion' of the laser substrate CO_2, i.e. a higher percentage of the substrate CO_2 in the activated form than the non-activated form.

c. **False** – although helium has been used as a peritoneal insufflation gas at laparoscopy, it is not appropriate, as an insufflation gas for laparoscopy ought to be highly soluble in water, which helium is not.

d. **False** – helium has a low density and therefore is appropriate for upper airway obstruction (e.g. in laryngeal oedema) where the obstruction is orificial. It is not appropriate for use in bronchial asthma (lower airway obstruction), where the obstruction is 'tubular' and therefore the relevant property is viscosity. The viscosity of helium is higher than that of air (nitrogen/oxygen).

e. **True** – because it will help avoid 'nitrogen narcosis'. Nitrogen narcosis is a specific example of the more general 'inert gas narcosis' relating to general anaesthesia. It is based on the theory that the size and thickness of nerve membranes determine their ability to conduct nerve impulses, and these in turn depend on the size and amount of gas molecules dissolved in them. Nitrogen, being a larger molecule than helium, will impair nerve conduction and bring about narcosis at a much lower concentration than helium. Therefore breathing a helium–oxygen mixture will enable a diver to descend to a much lower level (700 m) without narcosis than breathing air nitrogen/oxygen (only about 50 m).

5.55 Answers

a. **True**.

b. **False** – for Boyle's law to hold good the temperature must be constant, therefore the conditions must be isothermal, not adiabatic.

c. **True** – the Joule–Thomson effect is adiabatic decompression.

d. **True** – adiabatic decompression (see **c**.)

e. **True** – adiabatic compression, leading to a rise in temperature, can occur at the Bodok seal if a full cylinder is opened rapidly.

5.56 Answers

a. **True** – trifluoromethyl vinyl ether is better known as Compound A, which is produced with sevoflurane.

b. **True** – which was produced with trichloroethylene, an agent no longer in use.

c. **False** – acetone collects in the circuit because of release from the patient's system, not because of reaction of anaesthetic agent with soda lime.

d. **False**.

e. **False** – like acetone, methane is released into the circuit from the patient's system.

5.57 Answers

a. True – it may be described as the 'copper kettle principle par excellence'.
b. False – using 100% oxygen.
c. True.
d. True.
e. False – it accurately delivers the dialled v.p.c. (volumes per cent) of agent but when its gas is brought to ambient atmospheric pressure at high altitudes, the v.p.c. represents an absolute decrease in the partial pressure of the agent.

5.58 Answers

a. True – morphine on undergoing Phase II conjugation produces two metabolites: morphine-6-glucuronide, which is analgesic, and morphine-3-glucuronide, which has no analgesic action.
b. True – suxamethonium is broken down in a two-stage process first to succinyl monocholine and then choline and succinic acid. Succinyl monocholine too is a neuromuscular blocker drug, albeit a weaker one.
c. True – hydroxymidazolam, the metabolite, also has an action similar to midazolam.
d. True – deacetylation of vecuronium at the 3-OH position produces the major metabolite 3-OH vecuronium, which is nearly as potent as the parent compound.
e. True – the major metabolite, nor-pethidine, has analgesic activity (and is twice as potent as pethidine in inducing seizures).

5.59 Answers

a. False – primary action (+++) at H_1 sites; secondary: (++) muscarinic (M) and D_2 sites.
b. False – primary action M (+++); secondary: (++) D_2.
c. True – primary: D_2 (+++); secondary: 5-HT_3 (++).
d. False – sole site: 5-HT_3 (+++).
e. False – the site of anti-emetic action of dexamethasone is still unknown.

5.60 Answers

a. True – in the stomach a large percentage of the aspirin is converted to salicylic acid, which has a pKa of c. 3.5. In the acid environment of the stomach (pKa c. 2–2.5), most of the salicylic acid is in the non-ionised and therefore lipophilic form and thus capable of crossing the gastric mucosal membrane by simple diffusion.

b. False – is well bound to plasma albumin.

c. True – is converted to salicylic acid by non-specific esterases.

d. True – routine coagulation tests do not measure platelet activity.

e. True – the pharmacodynamic effect is the duration of platelet inhibition, c. 10–12 days. The pharmacokinetic effect is the duration of the physical presence of the drug in the body in its 'native' form, which is c.15 minutes for aspirin and c. 2–12 hours for salicylate.

5.61 Answers

a. False – aspirin does not inactivate lipoxygenase, the enzyme responsible for the formation of leukotrienes.

b. True – by acetylating the serine moiety in the enzyme by covalent bonding.

c. False – it is secondary to suppression of 'peripheral' prostaglandin production.

d. False – by forced alkaline diuresis.

e. False – the tinnitus is reversible on withdrawal of the drug.

5.62 Answers

a. True.

b. False – metformin is regarded as an 'antihyperglycaemic agent', because it does not promote insulin release from the pancreas, but: (i) increases the action of insulin in peripheral tissues; (ii) inhibits gluconeogenesis; and (iii) reduces intestinal absorption of glucose.

c. False – it is absorbed mainly in the small intestine.

d. False – does not bind to plasma proteins.

e. False – it is excreted unchanged.

5.63 Answers

a. False – if the electrodes are too near the muscle, there could be direct muscle stimulation.

b. False – a cooler skin will have a higher impedance, which will reduce the current strength in accordance with Ohm's law.

c. True.

d. True – the little finger muscles could be directly stimulated.

e. True – because of the need to satisfy the requirement of the all-or-none property of muscle.

5.64 Answers

a. **False**.
b. **False** – it is regarded as a pre-synaptic event.
c. **True** – it is also known as 'mixed' block and 'desensitising' block.
d. **True**.
e. **True** – but it is no guarantee.

5.65 Answers

a. **True** – presumably by blocking Ca^{2+} channels.
b. **False** – increase the ACh release at pre-synaptic motor terminals.
c. **False** – tetracyclines do impair NM transmission but by showing activity at the post-junctional site.
d. **True**.
e. **True** – by inhibiting cAMP release and thereby reducing pre-synaptic acetylcholine release.

5.66 Answers

a. **True**.
b. **True**.
c. **False** – binding to one α subunit is sufficient in either case.
d. **True**.
e. **False** – in the Eaton–Lambert syndrome the patient is 'sensitive' to both types of NMBAs. In myasthenia gravis the patient is sensitive to non-depolarisers, but resistant to depolarisers.

5.67 Answers

a. **True**.
b. **False** – because of the change in pH, it becomes less soluble.
c. **False** – it is the enol form.
d. **False** – disodium edetate, as a bacterial retardant, is present in propofol.
e. **False** – contains sodium carbonate to prevent acidification by atmospheric carbon dioxide.

5.68 Answers

a. **True**.
b. **True**.
c. **True** – it binds to the β subunit of the $GABA_A$ receptor and thereby potentiates the chloride current.
d. **True**.
e. **False** – the general anaesthetic and some analgesic effects are due to NMDA receptor interaction.

5.69 Answers

a. **True**.
b. **True**.
c. **True**.
d. **True**.
e. **True**.

5.70 Answers

a. **True**.
b. **False** – by hepatic biotransformation.
c. **False** – by exhalation.
d. **True**.
e. **True** – ketamine undergoes both redistribution as well as demethylation and hydroxylation by hepatic enzymes.

5.71 Answers

a. **True** – it is found in diazepam.
b. **False** – cremophor EL was an additive in propofol but was removed because of its propensity to cause allergic effects. Cremophor EL is polyoxylated castor oil: polyoxyethylene glycerol tri-ricinoleate 35.
c. **True**.
d. **True** – it is found with sodium hydroxide so as to adjust the pH.
e. **False** – sodium carbonate is an additive in thiopentone sodium.

5.72 Answers

a. **False** – it is the highest: 6.0. Halothane: 0.75; enflurane: 1.6; isoflurane: 1.2; sevoflurane: 2.0.
b. **True** – c. 23.5°C. Halothane: 50.2; enflurane: 56.5; isoflurane: 48.5; sevoflurane: 58.5.
c. **True** – 0.42. Halothane: 2.3; enflurane: 1.91; isoflurane: 1.43; sevoflurane: 0.69.
d. **True** – c. 0.02%.
e. **False** – it is the highest. Desflurane > enflurane > isoflurane. Sevoflurane and halothane are reputed not to form CO with soda lime.

5.73 Answers

a. **True** – obtained from *Erythroxylon coca*.
b. **True** – because it breaks down to *o*-toluidine, which is the definitive agent causing methaemoglobinaemia.
c. **True** – cocaine is also a vasoconstrictor but it is a naturally occurring compound.
d. **False** – all currently used LAs are racemates and are available for use as such except lignocaine (Lidocaine) and Amethocaine, which are achiral, and ropivacaine and levobupivacaine, which, though chiral, are available as their S-enantiomers.
e. **False** – ropivacaine is also available as a pure enantiomer (see **d.**)

5.74 Answers

a. **False** – the others show no ceiling effect either. The ceiling effect is essentially a property of mixed agonist/antagonist opioids.
b. **True** – the uptake for the others is: fentanyl: 75%; pethidine: 65%; sufentanil: 75%; remifentanil: insignificant.
c. **True** – c. 20–40%, compared with c. 80% for the others.
d. **True** – it produces two glucuronides, morphine-3-glucuronide, the major metabolite, and morphine-6-glucuronide, the minor (c. 15%) metabolite, which is twice as potent as morphine in its analgesic property.
e. **True** – contrast fentanyl.

5.75 Answers

a. **False**.
b. **False**.
c. **True**.
d. **True**.
e. **False**.

5.76 Answers

a. **True**.
b. **True** – it needs to be converted to morphine to exert its analgesic action.
c. **True** – 60%. For morphine it is c. 25%.
d. **False** – better.
e. **True**.

5.77 Answers

a. **True**.
b. **True**.
c. **False** – the mechanism of anti-emetic action of corticosteroids is as yet unknown.
d. **True** – droperidol is a butyrephenone and is a neuroleptic as well as an anti-emetic. It acts predominantly by D_2 receptor antagonism and to a slight extent on 5-HT_3 receptors.
e. **True** – metoclopramide is a benzamide that acts mainly via D_2 receptors and to a lesser extent through 5-HT_3 receptors.

5.78 Answers

a. **False** – by chemical antagonism.
b. **False** – by chemical antagonism.
c. **False** – by 'neutralising' the acid by increasing the production and viscosity of gastric mucus.
d. **True** – by competing reversibly with histamine at H_2 receptor sites.
e. **True** – by inhibiting the proton pump, H^+–K^+–ATPase.

5.79 Answers

a. **False** – inversely proportional to the BG partition coefficient.
b. **False**.
c. **True**.
d. **False**.
e. **False**.

5.80 Answers

a. **True** – the incidence is highest in females in the third decade of life; in males it typically presents in the seventh and eighth decades.
b. **False** – the weakness is in the proximal muscles and can sometimes be asymmetrical.
c. **False** – it becomes worse as the day progresses because effort brings on weakness.
d. **True**.
e. **False** – muscle wasting is not a feature of myasthenia gravis.

5.81 Answers

a. **False** – it is autosomal dominant but not sex-linked.
b. **False** – it is more common in women than in men.
c. **True**.
d. **True** – hence the total contraindication of barbiturates.
e. **False** – but it has been recommended as a therapeutic agent because the drug decreases haem consumption and thereby inhibits ALA synthase activity.

5.82 Answers

a. **False** – in about 5% of obese persons.
b. **False** – it usually arises in middle age.
c. **False** – more common in men.
d. **True**.
e. **False** – it is associated with morning headaches due to nocturnal CO_2 retention leading to cerebral vasodilatation.

5.83 Answers

a. **False** – the inheritance is variable and can include autosomal recessive and other modes.
b. **False** – the incidence is higher in children than in adults.
c. **True**.
d. **False** – a rising pCO_2 is more likely to be the prodromal feature.
e. **False** – there is a combined respiratory and metabolic acidosis, the former due to the rising pCO_2 and the latter to the severe hypoxia resulting from relative oxygen lack as a result of increased metabolism.

5.84 Answers

a. **False** – Mg is absorbed by an active process in the ileum. It is calcium that is actively absorbed in the duodenum.
b. **False** – Mg is carried bound to plasma proteins.
c. **True**.
d. **True** – at resting voltage NMDA channel gates are clogged by Mg^{2+}, thus preventing passage of ions through them. When the membrane is polarised the Mg^{2+} ions pop out to permit passage of ions.
e. **True** – magnesium deficiency leads to hypocalcaemia.

5.85 Answers

a. **True** – depending on the amount of $NaHCO_3$ that is infused. 8.4% $NaHCO_3$ has 1 mmol of sodium per ml (1000 mmol/L), an extremely high sodium content, and an osmolarity of about 2000 mosmol/L and therefore the possibility of a raised plasma osmolarity after its administration.
b. **True** – see **a**.
c. **True** – the alkalosis caused by the sodium bicarbonate leads to hypokalaemia.
d. **False** – alkalosis leads to a shift of the Hb oxygen dissociation curve to the left, thus leading to a lowered haemoglobin P_{50}.
e. **True** – paradoxically, the correction of the (extracellular) metabolic acidosis with bicarbonate can lead to an intracellular respiratory acidosis.

5.86 Answers

a. **False** – while carbonic anhydrase does increase the rate of conversion of CO_2 to $-HCO_3$ within the red cell, the reaction is not necessarily enzyme dependent. It can proceed without the enzyme, although at a much slower rate.

b. **False** – suxamethonium can undergo spontaneous degradation to succinyl monocholine and then choline and succinic acid. But plasma cholinesterase will markedly accelerate the breakdown.

c. **True** – NO synthase is essential for producing nitric oxide from arginine by converting it to citrulline.

d. **False** – atracurium is only partly broken down by plasma esterases. A significant proportion of it in the plasma is broken down by Hoffmann degradation: spontaneous non-enzymatic breakdown under physiological temperatures and pH.

e. **True** – dependent on cyclo-oxygenase.

5.87 Answers

a. **False** – enflurane and isoflurane are structural isomers of each other.

b. **True** – geometric isomerism is also known as *cis-trans* isomerism (see **d**.)

c. **True** – lactam-lactim is the generic term.

d. **False** – it is also possible where there are carbon–carbon single bonds, provided they are part of a ring structure.

e. **True** – a racemic mixture is a 50:50 mixture of enantiomers, which can only exist in the case of chiral compounds.

5.88 Answers

a. **False** – the strongest are covalent bonds: their Gibbs free energy (ΔG^0) is several hundred kilojoules per mole. Ionic bonds: c. 20; hydrogen bonds: c. 12–29. van der Waals' attractions: 4–9. London forces: even lower.

b. **True**.

c. **False** – although a predominant force in water, hydrogen bonds can also form between H and nitrogen (N-H bonds).

d. **False** – quite the opposite. The presence of van der Waals' forces renders gases 'non-ideal'. One of the criteria of an ideal gas is that there shall be no intermolecular attractive forces. Van der Waals' forces are dipole-to-dipole attractions between gas entities and their presence thus detracts from the 'ideal' nature of a gas.

e. **False** – London forces, regarded by some as one form of van der Waals' forces, are present in all molecules, even those that are regarded as non-polar. All molecules, even those that have no permanent polarity, can have temporary dipoles albeit for very brief periods (1×10^{-12} seconds), when most of the electrons in a molecule may be at one end. Their strength can vary from being much weaker than van der Waals' dipole–dipole moments to being about equal to them. It is the presence of London forces that makes it possible for non-polar substances such as methane and helium to condense to liquids. The London forces are named after Fritz Wolfgang London (1900–1954), German physicist.

5.89 Answers

a. **True** – they both refer to the cooling that results from sudden adiabatic decompression. Sir William Thomson was later ennobled as Lord Kelvin. Joule: James Prescott Joule.

b. **True** – the 'insulator' separating the two plates of a capacitor is known as the dielectric and may be air, oil or paper, or even a vacuum. The ease with which a capacitor can hold charge depends among other things on the nature of the dielectric, and this when compared with the ease with which charge is held in a capacitor in which the dielectric is a vacuum is the dielectric constant or the 'relative permittivity' of the capacitor.

c. **False** – an amphoteric substance is one that can act as both an acid and a base. Proteins are an example, so is water because it can dissociate into H^+ and OH^- ions. An amphipathic substance is one that has both lipophilic and hydrophilic moieties.

d. **True** – mho is the reciprocal of 'ohm', the unit of electrical resistance. Therefore the mho is the unit of electrical conductance, for which the SI name is the 'siemens'.

e. **False** – in channel-mediated diffusion the integral protein of the cell membrane merely provides a pore – a conductive pathway – through which the solute may diffuse passively through the membrane. It is *carrier-mediated diffusion* that is the same as facilitated diffusion. Here the solute binds to the integral protein and having caused a conformational change in it is 'facilitated' in its transfer across the membrane.

5.90 Answers

a. **True** – diamagnetism is a property inherent in all materials; some are in addition paramagnetic and some others are capable of the property of ferromagnetism as well.

b. **True** – provided they are at a temperature above 0 K.

c. **False** – helium is liquid at 4 K (the only gas to remain so) and therefore is used in the MRI scanner to lower the temperature of the conductor so as to render the material of the electromagnet superconductive.

d. **True** – glycine, the simplest amino acid, is the exception but it has no asymmetrical carbon atom.

e. **True**.